# Killing For Profit
## The Dark Side of Hospice

Michelle Young Doers, B.S., R.R.T., C.P.F.T.

Killing For Profit - The Dark Side Of Hospice
Copyright © 2019 by Michelle Young Doers
Revision 1/2022
All Rights Reserved

Copyright Notice - All rights reserved. No part of this publication may be reproduced, distributed, or transmitted in any form or by any means, including photocopying, recording, or other electronic or mechanical methods, without the prior written permission of the author, except in the case of brief quotations embodied in critical reviews and certain other non commercial uses permitted by copyright law.

No part of this book is meant to take the place
of sound medical advice.

Printed in U.S.A.

KDP ISBN 978-1-07441-281-4
ISBN 978-1-64606-054-2

First Edition 6/2019
Revised 1/2022

TheBreathingGirl@gmail.com

~Cover design is original art work by the author~
With the magic pencil given to her from her brother, Thanks John!

## Acknowledgements

There have been others along my own journey in healthcare that have helped mold me into the therapist that I am today. Without a doubt, they showed me, early on, through their own actions that integrity, honesty, and patient-centered care are standards to be maintained at any cost. I will continue to carry that torch.

BJ-Gave me my very first respiratory therapy position while still in college. You had more confidence in my abilities than I did in myself. You would also hire me a second time, thirty years later. You have been called home and are greatly missed.

VB and KL- Fresh out of college, you both pushed me out of my comfort zone, allowed me to fall, find my footing, and get back up. I have not looked back since.

LY-Oh, always the good cop! My best RT memories are those from under your watch. I have lost track of the number of times you rehired me after I left for travel assignments, dabbled in politics, or even to test the illusion of greener grass. No matter the situation, you always managed to see the bigger picture and the silver lining. Your guidance to all your staff members was priceless, and your management style was unmatched. You are truly loved by many, more than you know.

And as for SF, you left us too early, my friend.

Killing For Profit - The Dark Side of Hospice

Michelle Young Doers

It is easier to fool the people,
than to convince them they have been fooled."
— Attributed to Mark Twain

Killing For Profit - The Dark Side of Hospice

Michelle Young Doers

# Killing For Profit
# The Dark Side of Hospice

| | |
|---|---|
| Acknowledgements | 4 |
| For Love or Money - Love | 10 |
| Why I Wrote This Book | 12 |
| The Beginning of the End | 16 |
| What is hospice? | 19 |
| The Process | 22 |
| Ms. Minnie | 28 |
| Three Sides of the Same Coin | 32 |
| Quotas + Quotas + Quotas | 35 |
| What Ever It Takes | 41 |
| What If Your Choice Was Taken Away? | 44 |
| The Admission | 51 |
| Ms. Tacket | 55 |
| Welcome to the New Death Panel | 63 |
| Shortcuts and Systems | 69 |
| Mr. Voltz | 76 |
| Penny, Penny, Copper Penny | 78 |
| Mercy Killing? | 84 |
| Leadership? What Leadership? | 86 |
| Let's Talk Oxygen | 94 |
| Brandon | 97 |
| A Son's Mom | 103 |

| | |
|---|---|
| Don't Ask, Don't Tell | 108 |
| Companions | 112 |
| If It Starts Off Badly | 118 |
| Holiday | 127 |
| The Final Road Trip Home | 131 |
| Three Days Dead | 144 |
| Death Through Chemistry | 152 |
| Court of Public Opinion | 165 |
| Letter to Department of Health Services - Washington | 171 |
| For Love or Money - Money | 174 |
| Well, If They can do it,...... | 177 |
| Office of The Inspector General Report | 181 |
| Take Away | 182 |
| Further Explanation | 183 |
|     Ms. Minnie | |
|     Bedside Spirometry | |
|     GOLD Initiative | |
|     Road Trip Home | |
|     COPD | |
|     ILD | |
|     Death Through Chemistry | |
| Useful Links | 199 |
| About The Author | 200 |

## For Love or Money - Love

Europe 1944

As the outbreak of the Second World War began, Cicely Saunders abandoned her studies of politics and economics at St. Anne's College, Oxford, to follow her passion for helping others and enrolled as a student nurse at St. Thomas' Hospital. This decision would be short-lived. Constant back pain from a curvature in her spine took its toll on her as she performed her nursing duties, forcing her to quit her studies.

Then, in 1947, at 29, she returned to St. Anne's College, Oxford, to finish a degree in social work.

Working her way around the halls of Archway Hospital in London, she cared for a 40-year-old Polish-Jewish immigrant, David Tasma, who had escaped from the Warsaw ghetto. The waiter, who had no family in England, felt that his life was wasted as he lay dying. Their brief but intense relationship inspired the idea that she would help patients with life-threatening illnesses and provide a place for the dying to find peace in their final days. Mr. Tasma bequeathed Cicely £500 upon his passing in February 1948.

Almost two decades later, after finishing her medical studies, Dr. Cicely Mary Strode Saunders established St. Christopher's Hospice in 1967, the first of its kind. Dr. Saunders is universally recognized as the founder of the modern hospice movement, inspiring the creation of hundreds of hospices worldwide and cementing a new branch of medicine: palliative care. Dame Saunders' - Dame being the female version of Knight - legacy is too extensive and distinguished to be contained within these pages as she held over twenty honorary degrees from the UK and overseas. Additionally, to name a few, she was awarded the British Medical Association Gold Medal, the Franklin D. Roosevelt

Four Freedoms for Worship Medal, the Dame of the British Empire, and the world's most exclusive award, the Order of Merit*, by Her Majesty, the Queen of England.

She passed away at the age of 87 in 2005 at the hospice she founded out of love, St. Christopher's Hospice.

*Order of Merit - Established in 1902 by King Edward VII, admission into the order remains the personal gift of its Sovereign. It is restricted to a maximum of 24 living recipients

## Why I Wrote This Book

Just like healthcare in general, hospice has become part of the problem of elevated healthcare costs and decreased services. It is a business model built on cutting corners, making unkept promises, and placing the accountants' bottom line ahead of the care that the patient deserves.

These cutbacks have led to unsafe patient care with the wrong patient, wrong procedures, wrong medication, etc. The list goes on.

After over thirty years as a Registered Respiratory Therapist, I thought I had seen it all. I've helped babies into the world, and I've helped babies leave this world. I've spoken to dead people. I've witnessed death, helped death, and prevented death, all in the name of "healthcare."

Throughout my career, I have played a part in a patient's death and/or dying more than anyone else in the healthcare field or very close to it. I'm not talking about immediate death that comes from a tragic accident or the likes of a war. I'm talking about patients with prolonged diseases such as COPD, lung cancer, and ALS. Also, those patients whose surgery did not go as planned survived briefly, with the help of 'life support.' Or the accident victim, the near-drowning patient, the shooting victim, or hundreds of other ways people find themselves trapped in the healthcare system. Young and old, rich and poor, famous or not, I've treated them all.

Physicians and nurses may be the most recognized roles in healthcare, but the respiratory therapist is the life-giver and taker.

Whether it is called a ventilator, 'breathing tube,' 'life support,' or 'the Plug,' the respiratory therapist is responsible for the life-sustaining equipment. We insert the breathing tube when a patient cannot breathe. We adjust life support to keep a patient alive. And yes, we, respiratory therapists, are the ones whose job is to pull 'the plug.'

I spent too many years working in a field of treatment, rather than prevention, in a system that will explore every avenue to fight back death while trying to beat a disease. The whole person is overlooked in the name of treatment, and even at times, the patient gets lost in this fight.

To add to this, we all die. We may not want to think about it, but it will happen. While you may not have the choice of choosing to die, you do have the choice of how you die. At the very end of life, it is not that you die, but the way you die — I mean the last few months, days, hours, or minutes.

Will you die peacefully in your sleep? Most likely not. It will be a drawn-out process of suffering at the hands of others. And that moment may come today, tomorrow, or next week. We do not know the time and place of our passing, but you can safeguard the 'how' you die with knowledge of the system.

Somewhere along the line of human endeavors came the phrase "death and taxes." Shortly after that, I'm sure the first funeral service for hire was organized. And what comes before the 'death' part? The suffering. And so then came the service of hospice.

What a great concept! Everyone dies, so let's make money from the dying. But how can we maximize the dying process?

What if we could develop a business plan to provide services or the perception of services to the dying, say, in their last few months of life, and where there would be minimal chances of a lawsuit? And since dead people can't talk, and the families left behind just want to move on, it's a hospice win!

To be fair, the first hospices were genuinely concerned with assisting dying patients on their final journey through life, trying to ease the burden as well as the suffering while providing support to the patient and family.

Well, those days are long gone. Today, hospices are big business. And when I say business, I mean just like the insurance and pharmaceutical companies. Where accountants have more say in your treatment than your doctor, and your care is listed on their profit and loss report. You are just an entry in their ledger, listed as not a name but a number. And that number comes at the bottom of the page, on the last line and squeezed into the margin.

There will be stories in this book that you read and say to yourself, "No, it can't be like that" or" That doesn't happen here" or "Medicare would not allow that to happen." But I promise you, everything, and I mean everything, you read between these pages is true.

Why did I write this book? Because I came into hospice thinking, "What a wonderful service hospice provides, providing care and comfort to the dying." And then, like Dorothy in Oz, I found that behind the curtain of promises, it was all smoke and mirrors. The lies, the deception, the way services are promised and not kept. How medical information is manipulated to benefit hospice and how hospitals benefit from and encourage this behavior. Yes, unfortunately, this healthcare scheme extends into mainstream hospitals and doctors who also benefit from such practices while exploiting and targeting certain groups of our population.

Another reason I wrote this book is that, as taxpayers, we are footing the bill to pay for these over-inflated salaries and year-end bonuses for CEOs and other business leaders. They 'earn' these salaries and bonuses by exploiting every method to over-treat or under-treat patients through an incentivized system. Then, once they have exhausted the in-hospital reimbursement programs, they swiftly offload these patients to hospice care.

In many cases, this extra treatment leaves the patient worse off. And all the while, we are being short-changed.

I hope that those who choose hospice for end-of-life services will be wiser, know their rights, protect their rights, and insist on receiving the services that they are due and for the services they pay. I have seen too many patients and families who were misled and became trapped in a system that profits from their suffering.

Within these pages are end-of-life events, where you will learn how not to get lost in a system designed to maximize profits while decreasing care.

You cannot afford to wait until something happens to plan, as we are not guaranteed tomorrow. Today, we leave for school or work and assume we will make it home. Nothing keeps you from being one of the casualties of life you hear about daily on the news. You must prepare for the time when you cannot speak for yourself. And that may be just hours or minutes away.

Do your loved ones know what you want? Do they know how you want to be treated? Be prepared and take charge today for your final moments.

You deserve to know.

It's time someone told the true story about an industry that Kills For Profit.

## The Beginning of the End

I was out of state when my dad passed away in a hospice house. He had struggled with congestive heart failure (CHF) for years. My mom described the hospice house as having a hotel-like, almost spa-like atmosphere, with large, spacious private ensuite rooms and oversized bathrooms. Each room also had patio doors to a private screened lanai and a pull-out sofa for the family to stay in the room. Equipment like suction and oxygen was available, but housed in a decorative bedside cabinet, all within reach but out of sight. The building housed a community dining room, a quiet room, and an eat-in kitchen area fully stocked with coffee, snacks, and a refrigerator. Outside, there were picnic tables that overlooked a large lake. A fine hotel's trappings were present, but this "hotel" came with a very different price tag.

Shortly after my return home, I was browsing an online job board, searching for something different. I had worked in hospitals, worked for a travel medical staffing company, and worked in-home care, and now it was time for something different to expand my knowledge base. After thirty years in the healthcare field, I needed a change.

Looking online, I noticed that the hospice was looking for a full-time Registered Respiratory Therapist (RT). Up until that time, I did not know RTs worked in hospice settings. RTs, by training, are life-givers, not takers, or at least we try to give life back before we take it, but that's a discussion for another day.

I applied for the hospice position, endured two rounds of panel interviews, and accepted as the newest RT into hospice. I was the third RT in a relatively new program started by the hospice to have RTs on staff.

Since I would work for the corporate office, which "owned" two hospices encompassing four counties, I was assigned to meet one-on-one with each regional director of the two affiliate hospices.

The same inquiring theme arose as I made the rounds to meet these regional and area managers. "What brought you to hospice?" At this time, I would briefly recount my mom's experience with the passing of my dad. I also added that I was amazed at how thoughtful an organization must be to truly care about others, as having someone from Bereavement Services call my mom each month after my dad's passing to check on her. When they called, they would inquire if she was coping okay and if she needed a bereavement specialist to visit. Those monthly calls continued for about a year.

It wasn't until the very last director I met that the cracks in that facade started to show. But I did not recognize it at the time. It was an interesting comment or question from the director that gave me pause. However, I did not recognize it as an individual puzzle piece in the bigger picture. And it wasn't so much the question itself, but no one else who listened to my "what brought me to hospice" story said anything. I must have met with various department directors or managers to the tune of about fifteen between the two companies under the corporate umbrella. They all listened, patted my naive head, handed me a piece of candy, and sent me on my way. Looking back, they must have thought that we could mold another naive one into this culture.

And it came down to this very last director, who, at the end of my singing the praises and virtues of hospice with their monthly calls to my mom, that, looking back, this was the very first insight into hospice. It was like a breeze came through the room, shifting the curtain hiding all the secrets. She looked at me directly and said, "You realize we only make those calls because we have to, not because we necessarily want to."

I don't know if the shocked look showed on my face, but at that moment, my mind raced to recall the meetings I had had with the other managers since my hire. Did I miss something? Did I miss a word, a look, or anything? But my thoughts were interrupted as she shifted in her chair, "Welcome to the team, and please assist our admissions department as a priority."

This last sentence was pretty much what I heard from each manager I visited. What follows in this book are the stories of the patients I have met and cared for and the dim reality of hospice in today's healthcare system.

## What is hospice?

A hospice is not a place like a hospital. It is a health care philosophy with services usually provided in a patient's home, similar to home health care. It is an agency where nurses and aides visit the patients in their homes. However, we are led to believe that this service is specifically designed to meet the needs of dying patients. To be eligible for service, the patient must receive certification from their doctor or hospice doctor, confirming a life-limiting diagnosis of six months or less until their passing. End-of-Life Hospice Care

These services focus on a person's end-of-life journey. I call it a journey because, in essence, one travels from this life, surrounded by loved ones, into death. Death is the destination. However, as with all destinations, there are stops along the way, routes to choose from, and others to help, others being the living and the dearly departed.

In theory, hospice not only attends to the physical needs of the terminally ill patient but also the spiritual, social, and emotional needs of the dying person. As healthcare clinicians, we can sometimes lose sight of the fact that we are treating people. That person now becomes that patient: an ID band, an object in a bed, an interruption to our lunch, or an inconvenience.

Fortunately, predicting death is not an exact science; it is likened to a psychic with a crystal ball. Unfortunately, this foreseeing of death comes at an emotional price paid by the patient. I've seen too many patients whose doctor has told them that they have six months to live, go straight home, and start crossing off the days. Yes, counting the days. A calendar hanging in the kitchen, bedroom, or bathroom with a large X in each day's box, where normally you would find such items as recycle day, dog to groomer, or lunch with Betty Sue. These 'living' appointments are replaced with a countdown marked by two intersecting wobbly lines formed by red pens, broken pencils, or Sharpie markers. Sharpie markers are my favorite.

I have wondered what one does on the eve of their six-month prognosis. Do they prepare a last meal, watch old movies and lament days gone by, write notes of goodbyes, or lie awake all night waiting for 12:01 am as if to be visited by Jacob Marley and the ghosts of past, present, and yet to come?

And on 'that' day, what do they think will happen? A bolt of lightning will strike them in their easy chair, or some stranger will appear on their doorstep with a syringe and needle in hand, saying, "It's time." Or are they paralyzed by fear, as if blinking an eyelid would remind someone somewhere that death has not yet claimed them?

When six months and one day arrive, are they disappointed? Angry? Relieved? Or do they turn to the calendar and start marking the days that they have cheated death? Yes, that has also happened, but he started marking the days with a different color ink.

When I tell these patients that the 'six-month thing' is not real, they respond with either a confused look or "That's what my doctor said." Then it is followed by "Well, what does it mean?" Here comes the tricky part, where I sometimes wonder why I even felt the need to say anything because now we are at the 'do you want to hear the good news or the bad news first?' Like some sick and demented joke.

The 'bad' news is, in short, that you could have less time, or as some have stated, that is the 'good' news.

The 'good' news is that it is a rough estimate based on various factors, such as the diagnosis, overall health, and progression of the disease or illness. If you outlive your six months, the hospice physician can re-certify your six-month prognosis over and over and over again until you really need hospice services. Then, you will be discharged even though you actually qualify for hospice services. Discharged because you have been in service for five years, and a regulatory agency is scheduled to audit charts to ensure the proper guidelines for eligibility are being met, such as with Ms. Minnie, whose story we will get to right after I explain the process of hospice.

## The Process

As with any service, there are steps in a process that follow a particular flow.

Such as -

Referral to hospice
Education to patients/families of hospice services
Admission into hospice services
Discharge from hospital to home with hospice
Discharge from the hospital to a hospice house
Transfer from home to a hospice house
Hospice services in the home
End-of-life care
The dying process

Each admission into hospice starts with a process. The process begins with a referral, which can come from the patient, a family member, or the patient's physician. In the hospital, in most cases, it comes from the physician as a written order in the chart, and then that order is given to the case manager to contact hospice. A case manager, usually a nurse, is an employee of a facility hired to acquire patients when needed (fill the beds) and dispose of them when they are no longer needed (insurance benefits end). This is similar to how the human resource (HR) department works: acquire employees when needed and dispose of them when no longer useful.

Here's how it works.

A hospital's goal is to provide care to a patient until the patient's insurance and/or Medicare benefits are exhausted. The case manager's job is to relocate the patient when further care is needed. The service could be home care, nursing home, assisted living, or hospice.

Unfortunately, the patient's options are narrow if the benefits have been exhausted. With a chronically ill patient, hospice will be presented to the patient as the choice by the case manager.

The case manager will 'sell' the patient on the benefits of hospice, real or imagined, as they also outline the financial 'burden' that will be placed on the surviving family members if the patient does not choose hospice. The divide and conquer strategy involves engaging with the patient and family members separately to achieve the goal of obtaining an admission.

If the patient is hesitant, the case manager will arrange for an informational visit from the hospice liaison nurse to explain further (sell) the virtues of hospice.

The hospital's case manager will provide initial education on hospice and its services. The case manager takes vast liberties in explaining hospice. The case manager already knows your weaknesses, such as financial burdens, lack of family involvement, fear of dying alone, etc., and will use this information to sell you the merits of hospice and how it will 'help' you.

Basically, they are telling you what you want to hear so that you will choose hospice services.

To further solidify that hospice is the right choice, the hospital case manager, the hospice liaison representative, and the hospice admission nurse tag the patient as a team. Three white coats present themselves to you at different times, usually the day before and/or the day of discharge from the hospital. They deliver the same message from the same book, just read from another chapter.

You will have the hospital case manager saying whatever you want to hear because if there are any misunderstandings, the hospital case manager can easily blame the hospice liaison nurse.

Such misunderstandings as:

If the hospice liaison nurse's inferences were exaggerated, incomplete, or misleading, the blame shifts to the case manager or admission nurse.

And likewise for the hospice admission nurse. However, the admission nurse has more reason not to say or correct any information because their name is on the admission record. By this time, you believe what you believe, and he/she will not clarify anything for fear of losing the admission.

Using this three-person approach to 'sell' hospice, each representative in this triangle can say whatever they think you need to hear to get you to sign on the dotted line.

Also, during this emotional and stressful life-changing event, you will not remember names or who said what. You will remember the key points that were said or implied vital to you, whether real or imagined. You will not have time to think about anything, as you will be pressed for time to decide.

The hospital's case manager depends on hospice to get the patient out. The admission nurse does not want to explain why he/she lost the admission, thus not hitting their required quota and having the hospital wait or keep the patient. Hospice wants to help the hospital maximize the profitability of their beds and not "lose" money on financially strained patients. The hospital, in turn, makes referrals to hospice. Each hand washes the other.

The patient reluctantly chooses hospice. The case manager reports to the physician that the patient has chosen hospice. The physician then writes an order for hospice, which is signed, sealed, and delivered.

In some counties, there is more than one hospice company. The fight for admission is cutthroat. The race to be the first to admit the patient and gain that admission is paramount. If a particular hospice does not get the last referral out promptly, the following referral will go to another hospice. Future business hangs in the balance with each referral. If this hospice does not say the right things to get that patient into service and out of the hospital, they can forget about the subsequent referral. For hospice, admission is everything.

In some cases, the referral is made because the patient truly has a terminal illness with a life expectancy of six months or less. Those are the guidelines by which government agencies mandate hospices to operate. If you have six months or less to live, hospice will be there to help comfort and manage your symptoms during your final journey, your final chapter here with the living.

But what if you had longer to live and the referral was made based on a decision based on money?

What if you knew your doctor, the hospital, and the hospice had their agenda, and caring about you or your loved one's health and safety came with a price?

It happens every day. Lives are cut short due to monetary gains or lack of money in another direction.

Do you know what is covered under your insurance or Medicare benefits?

Do you know the benefit period and how long it lasts before it resets?

Do you know what you would be required to pay out of pocket on demand to continue receiving care at the hospital or long-term acute care (LTAC) center?

Let me tell you, your doctor, hospital, and hospice know precisely what is and is not covered. They know the reimbursement for the covered items down to the penny.

They are more knowledgeable about your coverage than you are, and they will use that knowledge to obtain every last penny of "care," "treatment," and "procedure" they can. When the money runs out, they are finished with you and will move on to the next victim. I'm not exaggerating.

The doctor's office is a business with a bottom line.

The hospital is a business with a bottom line.

Hospice is also a business with a bottom line.

And you, me, all of us are nothing but a line on an accountant's ledger.

Our healthcare system is now a system by which specific populations of society are preyed upon to make the rich richer - the hospital, the insurance company, the pharmaceutical industry, durable medical equipment (DME) companies, and now hospice.

The case manager will check a patient's financial situation to determine whether they can afford to pay the daily rate. If not, this is when the push to get the patient discharged happens, and the 'care' begins:

~ The hospital staff's attitude of - I don't care, they are dying/ leaving

~ Physician - Let's not worry about any more testing/procedures. They are dying/leaving.

~ Hospital bean counter - I don't care where they go; get them out. They are dying/leaving.

It sounds harsh, and it is—human nature. The patient has served their purpose for the hospital at this point. Everyone in this equation has an agenda, and the numbers overrule the patient— time to go. Given more time and aggressive therapies, such as weaning from continuous BiPAP, some patients could have had more time to live at home with loved ones. However, time is only given to the patient if you are like Ms. Minnie, who lived past her expiration date.

## Ms. Minnie

When I started with hospice, Ms. Minnie was a hospice patient, and when I met her for the first time, I was surprised at how 'healthy' she looked. Now, looks aren't everything, as we know. However, she walked, talked, and even went out to lunch with her friends once a week.

She lived alone and needed no special durable medical equipment (DME) such as a bedside commode, shower chair, or hospital bed, nor did she need any special medications or oxygen.

I would visit Ms. Minnie and do my assessment, including obtaining a resting pulse oximetry, bedside spirometry, and a peak inspiratory flow measurement. I would review her medications and medical history and then present my findings and recommendations to the hospice team via an electronic entry in her medical records. And to her credit, she needed nothing from me in the first few years she was a patient of hospice.

Over the years of my visiting Ms. Minnie, I learned - that she liked vanilla ice cream, did not want visits on Tuesdays or Thursdays (those were 'her' days), and wondered why a nurse would visit each week, or depending on staffing, every two weeks, to sit and chat to pass the time.

Of course, as the years passed, her health began to decline. By year three or four, I do not recall the exact year, her respiratory status required the start of low-flow oxygen usage, she was using her nebulized respiratory medications more frequently, and her breathing became more difficult.

By her fifth year in hospice, she needed to use a walker in the home. She was started on morphine to ease her breathing. Her oxygen was now at a higher flow, and she required the oxygen 24/7. It was at this time that the hospice physician requested I assess Ms. Minnie for recertification of continued hospice services.

When I last visited Ms. Minnie, I did not know it would be for the last time. She was to the point where she would leave her front door unlocked because she was too short of breath and did not have the strength to answer the door. Her medications, which would be delivered by UPS or USPS, would sit on her doorstep until someone came by to take them to her. She was short of breath just sitting there. Her sofa had become her daytime chair and her nighttime bed, with everything within reach.

Her eyes betrayed the smile on her face, showing that her life was slipping away as if in slow motion. She was tired, and just living was an effort. Her pulse oximetry reading on room air was 87% at rest, and her FEV1 was 16% of what would be predicted for her to do. She could only speak one or two words at a time without having to take another breath.

Ms. Minnie would be classified as a GOLD 4 (Very Severe COPD) and a Grade 4 (Too breathless to leave the house or breathless with dressing/undressing), which are assessments used by medical researchers to measure health status and predict mortality risk.

Clearly, Ms. Minnie was hospice-appropriate. The problem? She had been in service too long, and that would be an automatic red flag to any outside agency that would audit her chart.

So what happened? She was discharged. After five years of being in hospice service, she was discharged. Not only because of her length of stay but, I believe, because she was now cutting into the hospice profit margin. The cost came from DME equipment, aide services, medications, and an increase in nursing visits that she now required due to her disease progression.

Waiting in the wings to pick up Ms. Minnie was the newest hospice player in the area who would take any admission to solidify the need for another hospice by their admission numbers.

It was a win-win for everyone except Ms. Minnie.

And there are those that think, ok, so what? She still has hospice.

Ms. Minnie was at the end of her life now, dependent on those who came into her home. There was a trust factor. Now, she had the stress of the unknown. What will the new hospice do? Will they provide all the same medications? Who will come to see me?

Then, there was the issue of changing out the DME equipment. It would have to be picked up by one company one day and then delivered by the new hospice some other day. Delivery people would be coming and going.

The discharge nurse from the old hospice visited to go over paperwork, and the admission nurse from the new hospice visited to go over and have her sign documents for their service.

I don't know about you, but even if I have a simple cold, I don't want to be bothered with all that mess, much less if I am on my deathbed.

Like many patients, Ms. Minnie was used to gain profits for the company until the cost of her care outweighed the reimbursement. Then, she was neatly disposed of.

The take away is: get it in writing. During the admission process, all those documents you sign are for the benefit of hospice, not you.

Let me say that again: During the admission process, all those documents you sign are for the benefit of hospice, not you.

Ask about any reasons hospice might discharge you, who will visit you and how frequently, what medications are covered, and what other services are available (chaplain, social worker, physical therapy, etc.), and get everything in writing before you sign anything.

Please do not accept "Oh, we'll figure that out once you're home." That is the ultimate line used. Why? Because they know most patients will do anything or go along with anything to get home.

It is all about getting the admission and then disposing of the patient when they are no longer profitable.

Here's the thing with hospice: the family is usually so distraught that they hear what they want to hear, and the patient just wants to be in their own bed at home. Sure, hospice has nurses who can and will visit the home any time, but what they fail to tell the patient and family is that some or most days, they don't even have the staff to make a visit. And if you do get a visit, it is hours later, if not the next day. Promises are made to get the patient or family to sign up for service.

## Three Sides of the Same Coin

The first side of the coin is the hospital, which employs case managers to monitor the census of the hospital with a bed count. How many patients are in the hospital, how many are private pay, and how many are Medicare or Medicaid? Basically, how much money is the hospital making per day on each patient with a dollar amount assigned to each occupied bed. The patients that are paying the least must make room for a higher-paying patient.

When they say it's not about the money, it's ALL about the money.

The case manager will approach the patient and family about placement options such as nursing homes, rehab centers, assisted living, and hospice. The irony is that most of us say, "Don't put me in a nursing home." But when faced with a nursing home or hospice, most will choose the nursing home. Unfortunately, by this time, the nursing home option is either too expensive or does not provide the level of care needed. So, hospice turns out to be the only option. The reason the case manager will give all these options is to appear to allow the patient to make a decision and be on the patient's side. "Oh sure, I can look into that." The case manager would agree with the patient, only to come back later that day to deliver the bad news, which the case manager knew all along.

When a patient becomes what is known in the healthcare system as a "frequent flyer," that patient automatically becomes a hospice candidate. A frequent flyer is someone who is in and out of the hospital or emergency room (ER). Most COPD patients are in this category. Though no fault of their own, it's the disease, the medications, pneumonia, or even a simple cold that can land them in the ER with an admission.

The other side of the coin is the physician. So, while the hospital does not necessarily want these types of patients because they are costly, neither does the primary care physician. Physicians are graded on many things. For example, how many of their elderly clients and patient base population received the flu shot? Not only does the physician get an incentive to give the flu shot by extra reimbursement, but the ratio of patients who receive the shot vs. those who decline the vaccination will also go towards the physician's 'grade'.

Another incentive for physicians is their ability to keep patients out of the hospital or emergency room. Re-admissions (those patients who visit an ER or have a hospital admission within a benefit period) are one of the worst marks a physician can get when it comes to insurance grades and reimbursement. To a certain extent, this is understandable. In theory, if the physician is treating you appropriately, why would you need to go to the hospital so often and 'spend' the insurance company's money? However, this theory should not apply to chronic illnesses such as COPD. It leaves the COPD patient with few options.

Both of these examples, as well as many others, tie doctors to Physician Incentive Plans (PIP). Insurance companies and hospitals have incentives for physicians to contain healthcare costs (increase profits) by paying doctors 10%, 20%, and 30% monetary bonuses for hitting their specific healthcare targeted goals. By incentivizing doctors with money based on how much money they save, the hospital or insurance company, whose interest is at the forefront of the physician's treatment plan?

And if that was not enough, insurance companies and hospitals want your doctor to put their interests ahead of yours. You have doctors receiving money from pharmaceutical companies. ProPublica has a project known as Dollars For Docs that tracks payments from drug companies to physicians. These payments include promotional speaking, royalties, business travel, meals, consulting, gifts, and various other gratuities. ProPublica found that as the monetary amount paid to the physician increased, so did the individual physician's percentage of prescribing brand-name drugs. A 2016 report states that these physicians "were two to three times as likely to prescribe brand-name drugs at exceptionally high rates as others in their specialty." Examples set forth were:

A New Jersey physician "who received more than $66,800 from companies in 2014 and whose brand-name prescribing rate was more than twice the mean of his peers in internal medicating".

A Wichita, Kansas physician "prescribed more than twice the rate of brand-name drugs than internal medicine doctors nationally" who received $11,700 in drug money.

A Brooklyn psychiatrist "prescribed a much higher proportion of brand-name drugs than his peers... while receiving more than $53,400 from drug companies."

Now I know that some patients just love their doctor, and you think they are friends with their doctor. I hate to break the news to you, but that doctor you love so much only gives you the time of day because of reimbursement. Would they, if he/she was not getting paid, sit there and listen to your aches and pains? Not at all. I would ask those same patients, Has your doctor ever asked you over for dinner? Did they pay you a visit on their day off? The most you can say is that you have received a bill, a magnet for the fridge, or a preprinted birthday card reminding you to schedule your yearly checkup.

So now we come to the third side of the coin. The third side? Yes, the edge of the coin that circles both sides. Hospice is constantly circling the hospital, the physician, and the patients like a vulture looking for its next prey.

## Quotas + Quotas + Quotas

It's All in the Numbers

Those who have bought a car know the feeling of a pressured sales tactic.

> You need the car
> You love the car
> You want the car!!!

The salesperson knows that information and uses it against you to sell you that car at a price, maybe even a little higher than average. And the options... who can say no to them? Leather seats $1200, Automatic transmission $800, etc., and you need to protect that investment with the $5000 bumper-to-bumper warranty, or so the salesman wants you to think.

And the little extras they throw in to sweeten the pot: If your car ever needs service, you'll get a free oil change and shuttle service. Financing? Don't worry, we can take care of that!

But we know this about buying a car before we even step foot onto a dealership lot. Or, at the very least, you will after you buy your first car. It's a lesson you will not forget.

Now I'm not picking on car dealerships; it's a business, and we know that business model and how it works. They sum up your car, the way you dress and how you speak. They are making a mental profile of you regarding your income and education level, two things that will be used to their advantage to either sell you a higher-priced car or pay more for the car you pick.

The basic knowledge we should have about buying a car is that the salesperson has their agenda. With each car sale, the salesperson receives a bonus, commission, or some other incentive to sell you that car.

Now, take that same car salesperson and have them wear a lab coat. Has anything changed other than their appearance? Move this person from the car dealership and place them in a hospital at the bedside of your loved one. Has anything changed other than the appearance and location? Nope. Let me explain.

Hospice is a business. Even nonprofit hospices drive to make a profit. They have processes, systems, programs, and incentives to make a profit, with the majority going to the company's board, the CEO's salary, and the Vice President's bonuses, trips, allowances, perks, and incentives to allow them to keep their job. Because if they don't do it, someone else will.

The hospice representative standing at your bedside or the bedside of your loved one has an agenda. It can be summed up in one word: quota.

After a referral from the hospital is received at the hospice office, it will be assigned to a representative to visit the patient and explain the services offered and benefits of hospice. The representative may be a social worker (SW) or a registered nurse (RN). This is where the 'sale' begins.

You may not think of your healthcare provider or bedside nurse as a salesperson, but that is what it has come down to. They are selling you a service. And lest you forget, you are buying AND paying for this service.

You are not at the mercy of their 'services' even though it may be presented in a way that they are doing you a favor.

Healthcare, all around, is a business. What counts is making the money and spending as little as possible. The hospital's attempt to spend as little money as possible begins when the patient is referred to hospice. At that point, the hospital will do very little to help you. Remember, you are costing them money at this point. No more diagnostic procedures unless good reimbursement is involved. And you can forget about them trying to wean your loved one from life support or continuous BiPAP, because they do not want to chance the death on their records.

When I started in the field of hospice, the admission nurses were given gift cards if they made or exceeded their quota. Since then, when times are tough, now it's an expectation of the job. If an admission nurse works eight hours, they have a quota of 2 admissions. If they work twelve hours, they have a quota of three admissions.

If you knew the person standing at your bedside or the bedside of your loved one had a quota to fulfill, would you think differently about the 'services' they are offering? All those little things they tell you about music therapy, pet therapy, volunteer services, chaplains, aides to help several times a week, nurses who visit in the home, medications that will be supplied, 24-hour nurse on-call service, etc., really are only partially available or not available at all?

What the admission nurse says or implies is not reality. It is a shell game of what they can get a patient to believe and what the patient wants to believe; that when the patient chooses hospice, all the cares and worries go out the window.

They say you will have an aide three times a week to bathe you, but it ends up being one time a week. When one county has one aide, and the aide has 28 patients to bathe in a week, you will only have one bath a week, if that.

I always offer my patients a chaplain or social worker to visit. I offered the chaplain for months and received the same answer from the various patients: they had already requested a chaplain, but he was on vacation. When I brought the subject of the chaplain to one of the nurse managers, she flatly stated that the chaplain wasn't on vacation; he had quit, and they had not replaced that position. I guess it is just easier to say that the chaplain is on 'vacation' while that dying patient waits for his return than to say to that patient, "You'll be dead before we get a replacement."

Additionally, this is a very stressful time for the patient and their family. They are making life-changing decisions. And they are pressed by the hospital to make those decisions right now.

Think about that for a minute. How much time and research is spent buying a home or a car?

Are you buying a home in a neighborhood with good schools that will maintain property values? What's the MPG for that nice car, and what are the available options?

It may take weeks, if not months, to find the right home or car, but with life and/or death decisions like choosing hospice, they are very generous to give you until the morning to make up your mind. Yes, it's that cold. To them, it is cut and dry. You are a chronically ill patient who frequents the hospital, and they see you as a negative mark on their 'grade'. Any re-admission within that benefit period is a negative for the hospital and the attending physician. They will more than likely push you towards choosing hospice.

But some will say you have to have a terminal diagnosis of six months or less to live. While that is true, it is not always accurate. As with any industry, it's all in the wording. It can also be easy to describe a patient in one light or another. I have witnessed firsthand admission nurses giving reports to a hospice physician to obtain certification. These nurses are the hospice closers who are relied upon to get that admission. These nurses are the top producers of admissions to hospices.

For example, they will highlight all the negative items regarding a patient's health status while leaving out positives. When one such nurse finished her call to the hospice physician for certification, I asked, "Why didn't you tell him that the patient was able to sit in the chair this morning or any of the other good things?" Her response was, "If I told him those things as well, he wouldn't certify the patient." And the hospice physician? They accept whatever he or she is told. They know how the game is played and their role is not to ask too many questions.

Some patients manage to survive another day because someone else steps in. All too often, the person who could have stepped up to say something will not, for fear of losing their job. I understand mortgages/rent to pay, kids to feed, etc.

Or their attitude is one of-

"It won't change, so why bother?"

"Why risk it?"

"It's not my family member."

"It's their choice."

"You know how things are."

Yes, those are the answers I've received and many more excuses not to say something. Honestly, there are times I wish I was more inclined to 'go with the program', but I cannot do that. At what point do you sell your soul to be paid by the devil?

Patients cannot see down the road or around the perilous corners before them when discharged from the hospital. They rely on their healthcare provider's honest, professional care and advice to get them home safely. That trust is misplaced. Most, if not all, patients want to go home, and they will voice their wishes to the bedside nurse or the referral nurse from the hospice. That little bit of information is now used by the bedside nurse or the hospice nurse to the detriment of the patient. They have their agenda: the bedside nurse or hospital case manager's agenda is to replace that patient with a higher reimbursement-paying patient.

Much like a restaurant that needs to turn over a table, the principle is the same. Get the diner in and up-sell as much as possible: drinks, appetizers, mains, desserts, and another round of drinks. However, the after-dinner drinks will be politely offered at the bar. And when your money runs out, it's time for you to go, whether you want to or not. The restaurant needs to maximize every table. Numerous studies have been done on restaurant revenue management to help restaurateurs maximize their profits. The same has come to pass in the healthcare field.

However, you can choose your place to dine. With healthcare, you are stuck with where your insurance allows you to go. The doctor, hospital, lab/X-ray facility,... it's all down to dollars and cents, not about the care itself.

## What Ever It Takes

Mr. H is a prime example. One day, a PAC nurse called me regarding a patient at an LTAC (Long Term Acute Care). These facilities are "rehabilitative" for patients who are not quite ill enough for the hospital but still need 24/7 nursing care.

Additionally, these facilities are usually for patients on some type of respiratory support, either a ventilator or BiPAP.

This patient had a trach, and the nurse called me to inquire about what the patient would need at the care center. The patient is on "High Flow oxygen @ 21% with a trach collar."

It is humidified room air. There is nothing "high flow" about this set-up; 21% is room air, meaning no supplemental oxygen and a trach collar is a mask made for a trach. There is nothing special about these; the nurse is just getting information from another nurse about something neither of them knows. I do not mean to sound harsh towards nurses; it's just that it's not their area of specialty. This is why a whole profession is dedicated to respiratory issues: respiratory therapists.

Keeping in mind that these LTACs only get paid for so many Medicare days, once a patient has used all their Medicare days, out the door they go. They don't care where they go; they only want to get out of that bed. And the family that is told their loved one must leave is confused about why they must leave when they see empty beds. It does not matter how many empty beds there are if Medicare is not paying the facility to care for a patient. The facility does not want to pay the staff to attend to that patient. Again, it is all about the dollar. Not health care, the dollar.

So, when it came time for Mr. H's wife to be discharged, the same story was told to him like so many other families before. Facility rep: "We've done all we can. It's time for hospice." Then the hospice rep said, "Let's get your loved one over to our care center, and we'll figure out a plan." And, of course, that works. The facility is putting pressure on the family to get that patient out, and here comes hospice to the rescue.

I would visit Mr. H's wife at the care center the next day. As I approached the room, I saw Mr. H standing in the doorway. With his back towards me, I could not see his face until I was at his side, ready to introduce myself. It then hit me: there's a problem at hand. I could see the crinkled forehead, the flush in his face, the beads of sweat at his temples, and the look in his eyes that I had seen way too many times before. The look of confusion, anxiety, and anger. This is one of those times I wish I had a heads-up before walking into this situation. Whatever the situation was, it was not going to be good.

No sooner than the last word of introduction left my mouth, it all came spilling out of him, "I can't take her home, I cannot take care of her. Someone told me I would pay $500 a day if my wife stayed here. I cannot afford that. I told them at the hospital I could not take care of her at home". By this time, he was shaking with anxiety at the thought of caring for his wife. He did not know how to care for her. And his anger from being led to believe hospice would help when it was just a temporary one-night stay to remove her from the hospital. The confusion over what was happening. He was told that he had to take his wife home today or pay $500 a day for each day she stayed at the hospice house.

Mr. H, also in his late seventies, was at a loss. The medical system had changed so many times in his life that now it's all too confusing. He is at a loss as to what to do. He wants to desperately help his wife but does not know what to do. His wife is bed-bound, trached, and minimally responsive. She will need care around the clock. The care involves bathing, changing, suctioning the trach, and feeding via a PEG tube. She needs care as a newborn would need.

The hospice admissions nurse spoke with the husband and offered to help with the care and would transfer her to the hospice house. What they neglected to say was that she would only be allowed to stay at the hospice house for a short time before she would need to go home or be placed in a nursing home. That short time would end up being the next day.

Yes, this is the reality facing our seniors during their greatest need. Just keep moving them until they are finally home for the family to deal with, and the hospice profits from the patient.

It is a win/win/loss. The hospital wins now that they have milked the Medicare and insurance systems for every procedure they could bill, and as soon as that money runs out, so does the care. The hospital bed is vacated for the next financial gain. Then, the hospice takes over to "help" by providing the barest of services and medications. This leaves the family to care for their loved one with minimal help from outside the home. The patient does not die at the hospital, so the hospital's mortality rate stays low, and the rate of admission deaths for hospice stays high. Hand in glove.

Michelle Young Doers

## What If Your Choice Was Taken Away?

It was supposed to be simple. The healthcare surrogate decided to have Mr. Zak transferred from the hospital to the hospice facility. He was to be removed from life support and made comfortable. "Comfortable" is a healthcare code word. For nurses, "comfortable" in this situation means medicating the patient enough to keep them asleep until their death. However, since the report we received from the hospital was that he had been unconscious and non-responsive, the powerful sedatives going into his IV were probably overkill. As it turned out, there was a reason for the sedatives. But not a good reason.

I stood in the back of the room, waiting for the distant family members to say their last goodbyes. I say distant because, of those that were now at his bedside sobbing with grief, none of them had even bothered to visit this man in the last three months while he lingered somewhere between life and death. He had been kept alive by a life support machine, a ventilator, breathing for him. That machine you would see in the movies or on medical TV shows. One of those "you know it when you see it" things placed next to the patient's bed. An oversized, outdated ventilator is stoically doing its job of breathing for the patient. The bellows on top of the machine add drama, as you can see the breaths given to the patient and hear the gentle whirl of air as the column of bellows slowly rises and falls. Adding to that scene is corrugated tubing coming from the machine that is connected to a tube placed in the patient's mouth as he peacefully sleeps. To complete that make-believe scene, the patient's hair is perfectly styled, and the bedsheets are pulled up to their shoulders and neatly folded over.

I laugh now just writing this, as this is rarely the case and far from reality in today's healthcare system. However, it does make for pleasurable viewing of an emotional scene in the movies. Now, before me, this gentleman looked like he had led a rough life. The white patches of grey hair on his head almost glowed beside his dark skin. The week-old facial hair, the half-on, half-off patient gown, and the crumpled bedsheets added to the look that no one cared about this man.

Instead of a breathing tube in his mouth, this man's throat had been cut open for a tube to be inserted through his neck into his windpipe (tracheostomy). The corrugated tubing from the ventilator was attached to this tube in his neck. It is quite uncomfortable for the patient as any movement of the tubing pulls on the tube in the neck and against the walls of the windpipe, causing pain and the patient to cough. Have you ever swallowed a little something the "wrong way," and it caused you to cough and cough, trying to get the item out of your airway? Now imagine that little something is a foot-long sausage. That's the feeling of having a tube in your neck to breathe through.

So far, we have a ventilator and a tracheostomy. A PEG tube is the last item in the trinity for low-cost, high-reimbursement billing. It is a feeding tube surgically placed through the abdomen into the stomach. I've seen thousands of these types of patients who become used for reimbursement profits. These patients are called Vent 'em, trach 'em, or PEG 'em. Check, Check, and Check. The exact recipe is used over and over again.

And this man was no different. He'd fallen victim to the system of doing whatever it takes to get a reimbursement, whether or not you need it. The system left this patient confined to a bed in the same room, looking at the same four walls, dependent on someone else to turn him and bathe him. And all the while, his mind lingered as his body withered in a long-term facility. A mind trapped in a body that has betrayed him.

But now, on his deathbed, these family members (one of whom was his daughter and health care surrogate) have to have their last goodbye. I wanted to ask them, "If you haven't bothered to visit him over the last three months, then why bother now?" But I didn't. I stood quietly, like a fly on the wall, just observing. As my eyes circled the room, my gaze locked with the attending physician looking at me. Our eyes conveyed a complete conversation without saying a word. We had worked together for many years. We knew what the other was thinking, and the slight roll of his eyes told me he was thinking the same thing.

The chaplain approached the foot of the bed and motioned for the family to join him. A wall of people surrounded this patient, this man, who lay motionless except for the slight rise and fall of his chest in sync with the breathing machine. The chaplain reached out his hands to hold the hand of the person standing on either side of him, and in doing so, the others around the bed also reached out to the person standing next to them.

One elderly lady, the patient's mom, stood quietly by the door. Dressed as if ready for church, she held a small Bible and tissue. Her little pocket purse hung on her arm, matching her small stature. She had not said a word nor displayed such outward grief as the others.

When noticed by those at the bedside, they called for her to come and join them. She shook her head slightly, then lowered her head as if silently praying, clutching her Bible to her chest. The patient's daughter had been the most vocal and dressed as if ready for a late night of bar hopping. She again called for her grandmother to join them. "Maw Maw, come on, don't be that way," as if scolding a child. The lady at the door gave no sign of acknowledgment. Now, turning her attention to the chaplain, the vocal one quipped, "Oh, forget her; go on, chaplain." And with that, the room fell completely silent.

The Chaplin began his heartfelt prayer. As he spoke, you could hear the occasional agreement or "amen," as you would listen to in any Sunday morning service. Of those standing around the bed, the vocal one seemed to be the chorus leader in the "Amens" and "Oh yes LORD," but in a matter-of-fact way, not as emotional as the others. But we all have our way of grieving, and, for her, this must be it.

Then, just as the final "Amen" left his lips, the chaplain herded them from the room. The elderly lady standing by the door stepped aside to let the others pass. She approached the bed once the rest of the family left the room. She looked at the doctor and quietly asked, "May I?" "Of course," came the response, and the staff, standing close to the bed, backed away to give her some privacy. We watched as she gently reached her hand into his. She bent over to kiss his cheek and whisper in his ear as he remained motionless. After a moment, she turned, said "thank you," and left the room.

As the door shut behind her, the physician and I moved to the bed, he on one side and me on the other. As he spoke to the nurses about the sedation, I talked to the patient.

I always talk to my patients, whether they are conscious or not. I believe we hear and understand until just after the last heartbeat and maybe even a little longer. I adjusted the life support tubing and readied the ventilator to standby mode. With a nod from the physician, I placed my right hand in Mr. Zak's hand and my left hand on his shoulder. Bending over slightly, in a calm and quiet voice, I said: "Mr. Zak, I'm going to remove the breathing tube from your trach to make you a little more comfortable."

I felt a slight squeeze in my hand. Moving my hand a little in his hand, I asked, "Mr. Zak, can you squeeze my hand?" I felt him squeeze my hand again. I look up at the physician, raising my eyebrows. The physician motioned to me the question, "Did he squeeze your hand?" I gave a nod. The nurse immediately reached for the IV pump to provide the patient with more "comfort" sedation.

Sedation. Just the word reminds me of so many other patients who were either helped by a chemical relaxation process or were "helped" into a restful, never-ending sleep. One such medication used for sedation is morphine. Morphine is an effective pain reliever, and it can also help with symptom management in the respiratory-compromised patient. And yes, it certainly has its abusive properties alongside the possibility of overuse.

I encourage all of my patients to keep a daily ledger of their medications, including the following: what medication was taken, what dose (how much was taken), and what time. Additionally, it includes over-the-counter drugs, herbal supplements, and even vitamins and minerals that are taken. Also, on the ledger, place comments on how you responded to the medications.

It allows your physician to evaluate the effectiveness of the medications and any adverse reactions. For example, suppose you are taking any pain medication. In that case, it is helpful to your physician to know what the severity of the pain is on the pain scale of 1 to 10 (10 being the worst) before taking the pain medication, how much medication was taken, and the response of pain relief obtained with a re-evaluation of the pain scale an hour later. Also, keeping a ledger serves as a check and balance on your medications and allows other caregivers to know what medication is due and when.

The physician told the nurse no more sedation for right now, and then he touched Mr. Zak on the shoulder and called his name. Nothing. Again, the physician called his name and told him we were going to remove the breathing machine and make him comfortable. At that moment, Mr. Zak's eyes flashed open as wide as saucers as he tried to shake his head back and forth. "Mr. Zak, it's okay, I'm right here," I said as I felt his hand grip mine a little tighter. I looked at the physician and said, "Now what?"

The physician continued to talk to Mr. Zak to determine his level of understanding by asking simple yes or no questions that Mr. Zak could answer by nodding "yes" or shaking his head "no". And the conclusion we reached was that Mr. Zak knew what was going on. Once that was established, the physician finally asked the most important question: did he want the life support removed? He shook his head no. I gave the physician a look that expressed I was at a full stop and would not be moving forward with the withdrawal of life support. Clearly, this gentleman did not give consent.

Mr. Zak tried to pull his hand up, but he couldn't. His arm was tied down to the bed, obviously leftover from the hospital. What unconscious, non-responsive patient needs his arm tied down in restraints? I untied his hand. He lifted his hand to his neck as if he was going to try to cover his trach with his finger so he could talk. Trach patients learn early on how to talk as they become frustrated with others' misunderstanding of what they want or need. This told me, at some point, this gentleman was aware enough to learn this maneuver.

I asked him to hold on a minute while I changed him to an oxygen trach mask and deflated his trach cuff so he could speak. I told him I would take him off the machine for just a minute so he could talk, but then I would place him back on. He nodded. I disconnected the breathing tube coming from the ventilator where it was attached to his trach and held an oxygen mask in its place. I said, "Okay, Mr. Zak, you can talk." He took in a big breath, placed his finger over his trach and said: "Don't you all kill me."

And with that, we were finished.

Some patients can speak for themselves if given the chance, and others, not so much. The choices you make for yourself do impact your life, whether it is ending your life or extending it in one form or another. You must make your choices known, concisely, with expectations and exceptions. Please do not wait until something happens to try and backtrack with making those decisions, because most likely you will not have a voice when your voice needs to be heard. If your end-of-life decisions are not known, someone else with their agenda will speak for you, which may or may not be your wishes nor in your best interest.

Mr. Zak was being readied for transport back to the hospital. As I passed his room, I saw the nurses "fluffing and buffing" him. Which, for us, meant a bath, a shave, and clean sheets. It was probably his first care and attention in a while. In a way, I believe this was therapeutic for him and the nurses. He was receiving care and love while these nurses were doing what they loved and cared about, which was caring for those who could not take care of themselves. Maybe this wasn't a wasted trip after all.

The hallway was now quiet as I made my way to the parking lot door, except one lone voice coming from the quiet room. I recognized the voice as that of the physician in the room with Mr. Zak. At this point, he was telling the family what had happened and what Mr. Zak wanted. I placed my hand on the door push plate to leave. As the door swung open, I heard a slight commotion behind me. I turned to see the little elderly lady walking towards the parking lot door, her head bowed with a soft smile. Standing in the hallway, just behind her, was "the vocal one" with her hands on her hips, staring at the physician. She was visibly emotional now. Crying. Real tears rolled down her face, along with her overdone eyeshadow and mascara. She leaned towards the physician and, with a stamp of her foot, reminiscent of an impudent child, yelled: "Well, why did you have to tell him?"

## The Admission

Once the referral/educational visit has been made, now comes the crucial decisions.

The patient signs away certain rights, like the choice of a pharmacy, DME company, etc. It is your Medicare medical reimbursement dollar.

Following the 'sales' tactics used by the admission representative, another nurse will follow to admit the patient into service. While the referral/educational representative elaborates on the merits and services offered by hospice, the admission nurse will fine-tune the information.

Remember the example I used for buying a car? The salesperson would then broaden his or her pitch, potentially "overselling" the vehicle. The salesperson is free to elaborate on options, imagined or real.

The car buyer may ask if the car comes with a year's worth of oil changes. The salesperson knows they don't give a year's worth, but he does know that the first oil change comes with the purchase. But he'll hold that information, responding, "It's worth a try to ask." This will lead the customer to a false notion that it is possible. Otherwise, the answer should have been a flat "no, we don't offer that." When it's time to sign the contract, you are already "sold" on that car. Because they know people buy with emotion. You have already invested yourself in that car. When the sales manager arrives, nothing is left to do but sign the contract.

Basic psychology at work.

Buying a car:

As demonstrated by your arrival at the dealership, you already like the car.

The five senses connect you to the car during the test drive.

The salesperson can expand on the merits of ambiguous answers like "maybe" or "I think".

The salesperson leaves: the connection to/access to the car has been removed.

feeling of the car being taken away increased emotional needs.

You were left alone-to envision the car in your life, garage, driving to work, etc.

To bargain with yourself: if "X" isn't offered, that's OK.

The sales manager arrives—emotionally, the deal is already done.

Concessions on your part will be made, but that one-time oil change will be thrown in to ease the pain of the inflated interest rate.

Logically, you may not be happy with the terms, but you have already emotionally tied yourself to that car and are unable to walk away.

Healthcare:

You want help, as so demonstrated by your being at the hospital.

Uses the five senses: no privacy, noisy, not at home environment, hospital smell, lousy food, etc.

Hospital case manager-outlines lack of funding and medical costs per day.

The Hospice representative oversells the services that may or may not be available.

Physician agrees with hospice care - Feelings of abandonment and that care has been taken away. Increases the emotional need for help.

Left alone, he contemplates options. Envision yourself at home alone, unable to drive, bathe alone, or get out of bed without help. Hopelessness sets in.

Admission nurse arrives: You think you have limited options as outlined by the CM, real or imagined.

You are sold a service but provided the least amount of service possible.

While the admission nurse may again briefly review what the services entail, the initial hospice representative's description of services really sticks in your head, because that person told you exactly what you wanted to hear.

A nurse will visit, you'll have an aide, medications will be provided, and DME (durable medical equipment) will be provided, such as a bed, bedside table, shower chair, etc. Chaplain services, social worker, 24 hour on-call nurses,...

And here is the kicker: Unlike having a car dealership on every corner, some counties only have one hospice to choose from. It is a take it or leave it attitude because they are the only ones in town. The patient feels stuck with nothing, or at least something. The hospital is pushing for the patient to leave, and hospice arrives like a SuperHero to take all your problems away.

Unfortunately, your problems have just begun.

They know they have you. It's a matter of signing the consent.

## Ms. Tacket

Sometimes, it's not what is said but what is not said or the unanswered question. The implied, the unanswered.

Ms. Tacket, who has pulmonary fibrosis, was being treated at a hospital for respiratory failure. She states to the nurse that she wants to go home. Hospice is then called in to assess the situation. Ms. Tacket is on continuous BiPAP via a full-face mask strapped to her face. Continuous BiPAP, meaning 24/7, is qualified as "life-sustaining."

Think about that for a minute. "Life-sustaining" means it is needed to maintain life.

Now, while BiPAP will not breathe for the patient independently, it will augment the patient's breath. With little effort by the patient to breathe, the BiPAP unit will trigger a breath until a preset pressure is obtained. Then, the BiPAP pressure will drop lower until the patient initiates another breath. When the patient's next breath starts, the unit will again cycle to a preset pressure, helping the patient to breathe. As an example, if a BiPAP is set to 12/8 (meaning a high inspiration pressure of 12 cm H20 and an expiratory pressure of 8 cm H20) when the patient breathes in, the BiPAP unit will increase its pressure and flow to help the patient breathe in until the unit reaches that preset level of 12 cm H20. The BiPAP unit will decrease the pressure to 8 cm H20 to allow the patient to breathe out.

This cycle of a higher pressure and then a lower pressure continues with each patient's breath. The higher pressure eases the patient's effort to breathe, while the lower pressure splints the airway open.

It was about 3 pm when I received a call from the hospice admission nurse regarding a patient going home. The nurse stated that the patient was very anxious to get home. The patient was a 70-year-old female with pulmonary fibrosis in the hospital with continuous BiPAP in use. The nurse had already admitted the patient into hospice services, and medical transport was set for a 5:30 pm pickup. I asked the admission nurse what equipment was being sent home with the patient.

The nurse's answer was "On her home CPAP unit."

Her home CPAP, not a BiPAP?

When I questioned what oxygen was in the home, the response was, "I think she has a concentrator." "Think." "I think."

After seven years of working in hospice, you would think I had heard it all. However, every day, there's another "I think" situation and another patient suffering at the hands of someone who has no idea of what they are talking about or who turns the other way to an organization profiting from a broken system.

Here's the problem: CPAP (Continuous Positive Airway Pressure) is a unit that delivers one pressure. It is half of a BiPAP setting. So, using the previous example of a BiPAP of 12/8, the CPAP would only be one pressure, and it would be the lower number.

In this case, it would be 8 cm of water. Using a CPAP unit at night for someone in generally good health and for OSA (Obstructive Sleep Apnea) is acceptable. It acts as a splint to keep the airway open during sleep when the throat muscles relax. People who snore have a partially occluded airway. A CPAP unit helps to maintain an open airway. However, if the patient has other respiratory compromised issues such as COPD, a CPAP unit is not a good choice due to the constant pressure and the patient's having to exhale against that pressure. A BiPAP with the two pressures augments the patient's breathing, helps remove carbon dioxide from the lungs, and increases oxygenation in the bloodstream.

Additionally, in a hospital setting, the equipment used differs from home equipment. For example, oxygen. Oxygen in the hospital is pressurized. It comes from a liquid bulk system, piped into each room through the walls and pressurized air.

BiPAPs in the hospital use pressurized gases, allowing the units to achieve higher FiO2 (oxygen percentage). Also, these units are more adaptable to the patient. In the home units, oxygen is "bled in" from an oxygen concentrator or a portable liquid oxygen system. A maximum oxygen percentage achievable is roughly 45–60%, depending on the patient's minute volume (respiratory rate x tidal volume) and the expiratory pressure or bias flow. Also, oxygen from a concentrator is not 100%. It is closer to 85–88%. So, oxygen in the hospital running at 3 LPM is not the same as 3 LPM from a concentrator in the home. The hospital oxygen will have a higher FiO2 with the same flow rate as the oxygen in the house.

So here we have Ms. Tacket telling the nurse she wants to go home but does not know the consequences. Now, the hospice nurse will exaggerate the patient's desire to get home. Why? Because the hospice nurse wants the admission credit, and the hospital wants the bed.

Does the admission nurse bother to educate Ms. Tacket on the above, as we have just discussed? Of course not, because Ms. Tacket may rethink her decision and ask questions about the what-ifs and other options. Hospice does not want to discuss the what-ifs and options because that takes time. Time could be spent on having another victim sign on the dotted line, and then the nurse could place a check in the quota box.

I asked the nurse to hold that transfer until the morning when an RT could evaluate the patient for a safe transfer. The nurse stated she already had discharge orders from the hospital and that transport home was set up. Again, I asked the nurse what equipment was in the home, and she said she wasn't sure. I asked what the patient was using at that moment. She told me the patient had been on her home CPAP unit (brought in by the family). However, she became a little dyspneic, so they placed her back on the hospital BIPAP until the hospital nurse could give her some more morphine.

So, let me get this straight. The nurse wants to send this patient home on an inadequate piece of equipment than hospital equipment, which she cannot tolerate while still in the hospital, and the answer is to give the patient morphine. Huh? What?

At that point, I told the nurse we were not moving that patient until tomorrow when we could accurately evaluate her status for a safe discharge and confirm what equipment was in the home.

As healthcare clinicians, we owe it to our patients to educate them on all the choices they have before them and help them decide on the best and safest option for their situation. It is too easy for the nurse to say, "They want to go home." Of course, they want to go home, but do they know what that means? No.

Let's look at this another way. I have a driver's license, drive daily, and have seen NASCAR racing on TV. How hard can it be? They drive around in circles. I could go to Daytona Speedway, show them my license, and say I want to drive one of those cars. Now, being the professionals they are, what are the chances of me driving one of those cars? Probably nil. Why? Because I don't have the knowledge to drive in that environment.

Because what you see on TV is not the same as sitting behind the wheel of one of those cars. I don't know what I don't know. I don't know all the perils of driving one of those cars on a race track, but they know and would not allow me to place myself in harm's way... or their car.

However, we allow patients to place themselves in situations they cannot envision when it comes to health care. The patient knows a lot from their experience and what they hear from friends and family. However, they don't know what they don't know until it's too late. When patients say they just want to go home, it can lead them to somewhere they least expected it to be. So why is healthcare any different? It shouldn't be. We are the professionals. Our job is to do what is in the best interest of the patient's health and their choice, not a checkbox in the quota column.

As for Ms. Tacket, I visited her the next day at the hospital, and she was still in the hospital BiPAP unit with settings of 12/8 and 60% oxygen. When I spoke with her daughter, who was at her bedside, to confirm what equipment she had in the home, the daughter said she had a concentrator that went up to 5 LPM. This lady was going to need 12–15 LPM bled into a home BiPAP unit. And that little CPAP unit the nurse wanted to send the patient home on did not have a backup battery nor an alarm. For safety reasons, "life-sustaining" equipment requires a battery and an alarm. How would the equipment operate if there was a loss of electrical power? Who would know without an alarm if the patient's respiratory status changed? However, the admission nurse is not worried about what happens after the patient leaves the hospital; it is just that the patient has left. Sad.

I arranged for one of our outside vendors to set up Ms. Tacket on a ventilator but in BiPAP mode. A ventilator designed for home use with a backup battery and alarms. Also, liquid oxygen. No oxygen concentrator could come close to 60%. At least with liquid oxygen at 12 to 15 LPM, we might come close.

Had Ms. Tacket been discharged that day on that little CPAP unit with her 5 LPM concentrator waiting for her at home, she would not have lasted that night. And then perhaps that was the goal?

Over the next few weeks at home, Ms. Tacket was able to wean herself off the BiPAP to the point where she only needed it at night. This begs the question, if Ms. Tacket could wean herself off the BiPAP at home, why wasn't this done in the hospital?

Again, once a patient's financial situation or end-of-life choices are realized, nothing is done beyond basic care. The hospital does not want to spend more money providing services to patients who cannot pay. Even if you could pay any amount, once you become a do-not-resuscitate (DNR) or near end-of-life, it is time to go. The hospital does not want any deaths on their record, and for those deaths that they can see coming, they want that death to happen elsewhere.

While Ms. Tacket was home, I tried to check on her as often as possible. With the proper equipment, Ms. Tacket was able to spend another six weeks or so at home with her family. During one of my visits, her daughter Susan informed me that her mother had been seeing and conversing with relatives and friends who had passed away. I nodded in agreement, as I've witnessed this quite a few times throughout my career. These patients are in their twilight, not quite dead but not fully alive. Caught somewhere in between. These patients can be completely alert and orientated to their surroundings and, at other times, drift into a twilight world. In this twilight world, they can see and communicate with deceased family members and friends. Surprisingly, during and after these visits from others from the beyond, these patients become calm and feel comforted. They are no longer afraid of dying. It is as if the dead are there to accompany them on their next and final journey.

Some experts claim these "visions" are hallucinations caused by excessive carbon dioxide ($CO_2$) in the system, which is caused by low respiratory ventilation. Or if the patient is disorientated from sedation usage, such as with the use of morphine.

Some of these chemically-induced "visions" can account for patients who have hallucinations in which they pick unseen items out of the air floating in front of them, or they become agitated and "see" bugs crawling all over them, frantically swatting them away.

While these visions attributed to $CO_2$ or sedation seem similar to deathbed communications on the surface, when analyzed, they are entirely different. It is like saying bananas, and plantains are the same. Sure, they look the same, but underneath the surface, they are entirely different and have different uses.

With deathbed visions, there are recurring components.

-Visits from deceased relatives, usually close relatives

-Dead relatives are there to escort them to death

-Becoming aware of dying

-Welcoming, or at peace with, dying

-Overwhelming calmness

-Visions of lights, brightness, and "beautiful" colors

-Briefly, acutely aware of both worlds

No matter how this phenomenon is labeled—deathbed visions, deathbed communications, nearing death visions—cultures from around the world have noted these occurrences in both nonfiction and fictional literature for centuries. While scientists try to explain away these events, it would be utterly egotistical of us to think we have the knowledge and understanding to interpret them.

Ms. Tacket had mentioned to her daughter, Susan, that a relative had been visiting her. Susan, did not think much about it until she heard her mom crying out, frantic with fear. She went into her mom's room to console her, but her mom kept crying for her granddaughter. Susan tried to tell her mom that Catie was at home with Nancy (Ms. Tacket's other daughter), but Ms. Tacket would not calm down.

Finally, after a few minutes, Susan called her sister and asked about Catie. At first, Nancy thought Catie was in the living room watching TV. But she was not there. Now, Nancy became alarmed and began to search the house, calling out Catie's name. Still on the phone, Susan listened as Nancy screamed Catie's name, and her mom would yell frantically each time. Finally, Nancy found Catie in the middle of the pool, barely clinging to a half-inflated pool ring, crying from fright.

Susan turned to tell her mom what had happened, but her mom was now asleep. Peacefully forever asleep.

## Welcome to the New Death Panel

Healthcare is no different in its business model than any other industry. And that model is to provide something and make as much profit as possible. Part of that model is networking with other companies within proximity of the individual company to expand its customer base, keep up with trends, and squeeze out any competition.

All available healthcare options should be made clear without conflict or passive intimidation.

Would you ever think that the hospital or doctor you visit all have a hand in each other's business? And do they share the profits and losses of these businesses?

Let me explain how one particular hospice works with a hospital to monopolize patients within a geographical area, purposefully alienate competition, influence the patient's choice of providers, and jeopardize patient safety.

Monopoly is a great game that I played numerous nights as a teenager. However, in the patient care arena, it is no game. Or is it? There is your property (body), the money (yours and insurance), and there is a winner (them).

Is it a conflict of interest when a hospital's CEO is also on a local hospice's board of directors?

Is it a conflict of interest when a palliative doctor at the same hospital is also the medical director of a hospice?

Is it a conflict of interest when a funeral home is on the board of directors of a hospice?

Is it a conflict of interest when a DME (durable medical equipment) company is the hospice's sole provider?

Now, put all of those things together. Everything is stacked against you getting the care you deserve and need.

The hospital CEO's job is to operate the hospital in the best interest of the hospital. When that same CEO is also on the board of directors of a hospice, guidance will be given to sway the hospice's direction and service towards the betterment of the hospital. This happens as the hospital and hospice work together to meet their end goal, not yours.

The hospice benefits from having a direct line of admissions from that hospital. The patient can request another hospice if one is available in their area. Still, the system is set up to limit the number of hospitals and hospices within a given geographical area.

What if the state required a corner store like Circle K to prove it was needed? This means that during this time, a competitor could monopolize an area, price items at whatever the market would bear, open whenever, and sell whatever products they wanted. We would not allow that. But why do we allow that with our healthcare?

When a patient does request another hospice, the other hospice is given unrealistic demands for a fast discharge by the hospital. When that hospice cannot deliver, they are back to the original hospice that the hospital wanted to use.

If the patient is given a list of providers, the subtle flick of the pen or slight of the eye tells the patient which hospice to choose.

Now, throw in the palliative care doctor who works at that same hospital and is the medical director for the hospice. The doctor has patients in the hospital who do not have insurance, are demanding patients, or whose Medicare days within a benefit period are all used up. The patient is too poor to pay for services or is uneducated in the healthcare system.

The palliative doctor has been treating the patient at the hospital. Now, it's time for that patient to be discharged. That physician may suggest hospice. While the doctor may or may not directly tell the patient that he is the medical director of a particular hospice, when it's time to make that decision, the case manager will make sure the patient knows. The inference will be made that you will receive "better" care because he's your doctor, only to discover that you are now under the care of a hospice team physician who does not know you from Adam.

Imagine these three players sitting around a table having a friendly chat. Are they talking about sports? Weather? No, the hospital CEO is complaining about the patients cutting into their length of stay (LOS) statistics and profit margins. The physician is complaining about the patients who can not pay for his time or the wealthy patients who are too demanding. The hospice director is bending over backward to get all of these patients, whether they need hospice or not. And here's the kicker: the hospital and doctors will gladly transfer these patients from their care.

Let's take it one step further. What if a funeral home was also on the hospice board of directors? Now, four business members are chatting about increasing their profits and getting the patient discharged. Because four members of the business community will do what is in the patient's best interest, right? I will go so far as to say that these "pillars of the community" will conspire to map out your destiny. An overall system that they will continually tweak to meet their financial gains.

Once you enter this type of hospital system, you cease to exist as Ms. Smith, a mom with three grown children and grandkids on the way. You are now medical record number 5824791. You may enter the hospital through the front doors, but you will leave on a stretcher through the back doors to hospice. Then, from hospice to the funeral home. They have you, will use you, and then dispose of you.

I can see it as clearly as day. And if it is happening at this hospital, it is happening at hundreds of other hospitals nationwide and worldwide.

As if that were not enough, the final piece of that puzzle would be the DME company. The hospice has a contract with a DME company to be its sole provider. And they know that you have not done your research. You don't know what to expect or what equipment is available until weeks or months later, when it's too late. Which means you don't know what you don't know.

To keep the cost to a minimum, patient safety is sacrificed. For patients requiring continuous BiPAP usage outside of the hospital, such as at a hospice care center or the patient's home, regular home-use BiPAPs would be supplied. As discussed earlier, continuous BiPAP usage is considered "life-sustaining," requiring a backup battery and alarms. Ventilators are not supplied to patients of this type. Furthermore, the manufacturers of these regular home-use BiPAPs do not recommend 24/7 usage, nor are they FDA-approved for use in such a manner.

When I asked one in-home hospice medical equipment provider if they used regular BiPAPs instead of ventilators, the response was, "We don't supply ventilators; we use regular BiPAPs." I replied, "You know, you are not supposed to use those in that manner." "Yeah, but they don't live that long."

And if hospice is so negligent about life support, think about that hospital bed that is delivered by hospice.

I was in an elderly couple's home. The wife was taking care of her husband. The man was bed-bound in a hospital bed the DME company had provided. The bed was out of the 1950s, though they are still readily available today. This bed was a manual bed. A crank is used to adjust the head of the bed or the feet. This crank would be located at the foot of the bed, attached to the bottom of the footboard. How is an 80-year-old going to be able to bend over and "crank" the bed up or down into position, not once but numerous times a day? I looked at that bed crank as if it was an alien-"What the heck?".

I called the manager of the DME company and explained the situation. He said, "That's what they ordered, and that's what we delivered. We are not paid to think."

I stated that this bed would not work for this patient and that it would need to be switched out with an electrical bed. "Sure, but 'they' don't want to use them; they are more expensive."

And to go with that manual bed, delivered by a person who's "paid not to think," is a used mattress. A mattress that has been used in hundreds of different types of homes, with too many to count bodies on them-bodies that are bleeding, urinating, having bowel movements, vomiting, and other bodily fluids, all on the confines of that twin-size mattress.

But wait, you say, "That mattress has a plastic cover on it."
Why yes, it does.

However, that cover has a long zipper that would allow fluids to seep into the mattress core. "Well, surely they clean the mattress."

The "paid not to think" person will bring that hazmat mattress back to their warehouse and do a quick wipe down, only to have it delivered to you to use. And that mattress, with its plastic cover, has been loaded on a truck, drug upstairs, down walkways, through narrow doorways, wrangled on a metal bed frame, left in bug-infested homes, abused by patients and family members with items left on the bed and in the bed, all with the possibility of poking holes in that plastic cover that no one will notice. And then delivered to you to use.

When a family complains about the smell of the mattress, it will either be replaced with another or told they do not have a replacement. By then, their loved one arrives, and that smell is pushed to the side because now they have no choice but to keep it.

Sad, sickening, and scary, but true.

## Shortcuts and Systems

Hospice employees come and go faster than anyone can keep up. One reason is that this healthcare field is mentally draining: caring for those patients you so desperately want to help. The other reason is the physical, unrealistic demands and expectations placed on the employee. Vacant positions are sporadically filled, then vacant again. Vacant positions are posted on job boards with no real intent to fill them. Posting vacant positions on the job boards at least gives the impression of an organization making an effort.

No one person has all the pieces. The more you know, the more likely you will be disposed of. It's like a shell game, keeping employees off-balance and allowing the organization to keep services to the patients to a minimum.

It's easy and convenient for service messages to become lost when patients don't receive consistent care. When a patient does not have consistent care from the same nurse or team of nurses, it is easy for service messages to get lost. The fewer services the organization provides, the more money it makes. Your nurse, who promised you an aide visit, may be off tomorrow. The message was given to the manager but then conveniently misplaced or forgotten. The patient will ask again for XYZ to the next new face who visits, and the request may be fulfilled by the fourth week.

It is the same with medications, physician visits, nurse visits, and the chaplain or social worker. The patient tries to be patient and compliant because they want to keep the services, but they do not realize they hold the upper hand. The patient is paying for a service. A hospital, home care, or hospice is not doing the patient a "favor." The patient is doing them a favor by employing them as a service provider.

Unfortunately, when hospices have a monopoly on a service area, and the insurance providers dictate when and where you can receive services, the patient is left to the mercy, if any is ever shown, of the area where the patient lives or seeks service.

The outdated method of a Certificate of Need is entirely useless other than to serve as a way for organizations to gain a monopoly in a given area. Healthcare, in general, should be an open choice. Patients, families, and taxpayers deserve to choose where, who, and how services are provided. Why is one organization allowed complete control of services in an area? We expect free and open trade in every area except for healthcare. Why? Because we have been programmed to accept it.

Hospice will rush to get patients home from the hospital as soon as possible. Why the rush? Remember that the most essential thing to hospice is admission; admission starts with having a good relationship with a hospital. The "good" relationship depends on the ability to get the patient out of the hospital when the hospital dictates, not when it is safe for the patient. So practically anything is done to keep the hospital "happy" to keep the referrals coming in, and the patient is on the losing end.

Can you imagine having pain that was treated in the hospital every four hours with medications, only to be discharged home without any pain medication? Does your pain magically go away? Not at all. You have to wait until the hospice physician orders it and it can be delivered. And now, to save money, rather than having a pharmacy driver deliver these medications, they are mailed. Yes, sent through the US postal service to your mailbox out by the street or delivered and left on the doorstep by UPS or FedEx several days later. These medications will range from morphine for pain to Xanax for anxiety and breathing.

Each patient admitted into hospice service may also receive a small box of backup medications. This box, usually kept in the patient's refrigerator, contains various medications should a medical crisis occur. The essential comfort box includes medications for pain, anxiety, nausea, insomnia, and constipation. A second box may also be placed in the home with specific medications for the patient's diagnosis.

Do not rely on a hospital staff member or a hospice worker to have the items you may need once discharged from the hospital. Before you agree to be moved, have a family member or friend check to see what has been delivered.

What items are in the home? Do not accept "That will be delivered once you get home." Because once home to you may mean within hours or the next day, while to the nurse, it usually means within the week.

How about being sent to an understaffed hospice home? What could happen there?

Understaffing has a domino effect that cascades from one shift to the next, pushing patients to the side. Nurses complete a new patient assessment, which includes taking the patient's medical history, a physical evaluation, and planning their care. And when they don't have time to enter the information into the patient's chart, the information is passed on to the next shift. This next nurse is expected to enter that information into the patient's chart as if she had completed the assessment. That is falsifying a Medicare document, which is illegal.

Additionally, the nurses could lose their state-issued licenses. Also, how does the second nurse know how accurate any information she enters under her nursing credentials is? True.

While that nurse is entering information into the computer system from the previous shift, no one notices that you or your loved one passed away alone at 9 p.m., only to be discovered eight hours later at 5 a.m. When the funeral home complained that they should have been called earlier to pick up the body, the nurse blamed it on the phantom family in the room who wanted to spend more time with their loved one. True.

Certain medications and equipment require a doctor's signature. The doctor's signature validates the need for the medication or equipment and its appropriateness for use on a particular patient. The physician must weigh the benefits against potential harm regarding the use of all medications, as even aspirin has its drawbacks.

Likewise, medical equipment must be chosen so as not to cause harm, further damage, or even death. Not only does a ventilator provide increased ventilation (as the name implies) to remove carbon dioxide from the body, but it also regulates oxygen within the body and the body's pH (acidity or alkaline), all of which impact other parts of the body, including the heart and brain.

Life-sustaining equipment, such as ventilators, has its place. Extreme care must be given to the appropriate use, mode, and settings specific to each patient and proper interface choice. When it comes to life-sustaining equipment, there is no one-size-fits-all. The mode/settings/interface used to sustain an ALS patient will be vastly different than that of a COPD patient. Both will be different from that of a CHF patient or a pulmonary fibrosis patient... the list goes on.

So when a nurse needs an order, they forge the signature of a physician, or say, an ARNP who is on vacation. Why wait when the nurse has a pen in her hand? And when it concerns life support equipment like a ventilator and an outside vendor, who would ever know? True.

Except when the ARNP (nurse practitioner) is contacted to clarify orders she had written for a ventilator and the ARNP states she was on vacation and did not sign that order, you can imagine my surprise. Not only was an order submitted by someone other than a physician but it was also submitted with a forged signature. True.

Submitting such an order took a lot of nerve on someone's part. If you are bold enough to sign someone else's signature on a piece of life-sustaining equipment like a ventilator, what else are you willing to do?

This system of maintaining a relationship with a hospital extends to the relationship between hospice and community doctors.

It is illegal for patients not to be given the right to maintain their choice of physician. Even when admitted to hospice, the patient has that right. Or do they?

Patients would routinely not be told that they have the choice to keep their physician or that it would be presented in such a way that it would benefit the patient. As noted elsewhere, the patient would be admitted under the hospice physician services, but then, within a day or two, the service would be transferred to a nurse practitioner. But this deception goes further. Community physicians would remain the patient's attending physician when admitted to hospice so they could continue to bill for their services even though they would never see that patient again. And why would a hospice participate in this type of illegal activity? Because, as one hospice physician stated concerning this activity —"... a good referral source". True.

How many patients are admitted to hospice for end-of-life service, and the hospice physician who certifies that patient for service also signs a capacity statement for a patient they haven't even seen or spoken to? Too many. How would that doctor or any doctor be able to certify capacity for a patient they haven't assessed in person? ESP? Crystal ball? True.

How about the pediatric patient being sent home from the hospital? The hospice doctor's concern was primarily about the medications that were "discontinued, too expensive" or "can keep, that's cheap." I'm pretty sure he would not rationalize administering medications to his child in such a manner. True.

Billing for services and the coercion of a patient's family to deplete the patient's assets to qualify for Medicaid. The chart notes that the "family is not cooperating with the depletion of assets." If hospice can not get your money, they have no problem putting their hand in the taxpayer-funded social program cookie jar. True.

How many "truths" must be stated before this industry is ratified?

There are systematic approaches to 'hiding' patients from inspecting agencies.

These agencies inspect hospices and assure them they are operating within the guidelines mandated by Medicare. However, as with any industry, these agencies will only be given the information that hospice wants them to know, not necessarily the relevant information.

When 3% of hospice patients have been in service for two years, possibly up to five or six years, this information will be unavailable to inspection agencies.

There are several methods by which a hospice will shield the full admission time of a patient.

1. After five to six months, the patient is discharged and readmitted to service.

2. The patient is discharged from the team and admitted to a hospice house.

3. The patient is discharged from one team and admitted to another team within the same hospice.

By discharging, the hospice starts a "new" chart. Thus, the other admission and discharge are separate and "hidden."

And I'm only scratching the surface of how hospice organizations game the system.

## Mr. Voltz

The most vulnerable groups in our society do not have a voice, and hospice takes full advantage of such groups. The entire healthcare system knows it holds the upper hand, and it uses it against the pockets of society within our communities. These are perceived as disposables—the easiest to prey upon. They provide the organization with a means to an end.

One group involves people experiencing poverty with nowhere else to turn, as with Mr. Voltz.

Mr. Voltz lived in a small room that looked like it had been added to the end of a mobile home. His bedroom door opened with just enough space to squeeze past his twin-size mattress adjacent to the door.

Then, to the left of the door was a table that held his TV and nebulizer, with his oxygen concentrator on the other side of the table. A large electrical panel was across from the oxygen concentrator and at the foot of his bed. Yes, the room must have been a maximum of an 8x8 room. And to round out this living arrangement, there was another person who lived in the front part of the trailer and smoked in bed.

Now, I don't claim to be a genius, not all the time anyway. However, seeing something wrong with this set-up on several levels would not take a genius.

I emailed the team and social worker, asking the social worker to visit to see if any community partners would help with his living situation. The email I received back from the social worker stated that he had called the patient earlier in the week and that the patient did not mention any needs.

At what point in the evolution of the human brain did most lose the ability to use common sense? How can you assess a patient and their living conditions over the phone?

And hospice does not want to know. Otherwise, they may have to use man-hours to help the patient, relocate him/her, or report to various outside agencies seeking assistance, etc. The man does not complain and doesn't need much, and hospice collects the reimbursement for this patient each and every day. Why mess up a good thing?

## Penny, Penny, Copper Penny

Penny was in her late 40s with end-stage COPD. She lived alone in an older mobile home, dependent on her neighbors for help. She was admitted into hospice service with the use of a BiPAP at night and 24/7 oxygen usage via a nasal cannula at 6 liters per minute. She could barely reach the bathroom without becoming severely short of breath. Then, upon returning to her bed, she would flop down and immediately use her BiPAP for relief.

And she smoked cigarettes.

Now, let me pause and state that at this stage of COPD with a long history of smoking, it does not matter whether she stopped smoking or not. It would not change the fact that she was nearing the end of her life. If anything, trying to stop smoking at this point would be mentally and physically stressful. It was probably the one thing in her life that she could turn to, and it was always there.

I'm going to liken it to brownies. When I'm on my deathbed and ask for a brownie, don't bring me just one brownie or tell me how it will raise my blood sugar. Hopefully, someone will bring the whole pan of brownies so I can have some of the crunchie edge parts and the gooey middle. And I want to smell them baking.

What is essential is to smoke safely, which means turning the oxygen off, removing the nasal cannula, and going outside the home to smoke. Because of her living arrangements, Penny did not have that option.

Here, we have a lady scared that she is dying. She's alone, barely able to move from her bed, short of breath all the time, and completely dependent on others for food, water, everything.

And now, in the last weeks of her life, after a hospital visit, she is sent home dependent on a ventilator via a full-face mask (a mask that covers the nose and mouth) for nearly twenty-four hours a day. She is only able to remove it for long enough to go to the restroom or smoke a cigarette. A patient, at this stage, is not going to magically stop smoking.

Smoking is an addiction. But that wasn't hospice's concern. Their concern was gaining the admission and having the patient sign a "smoking waiver."

It did not matter that the patient lived alone, basically bed-bound, with 24/7 oxygen usage, and smoked in the back bedroom of a mobile home, which, in itself, was a disaster waiting to happen.

And it would not be the first time for hospice, as they already had a history of a patient who was in a similar situation. However, the patient managed to set the house on fire by falling asleep while smoking and killing her husband. Then, later, another fire killed her. But I'm sure there was a smoking waiver in place.

Penny was alone as I walked into her home. From the outside, it looked like an old abandoned trailer, but inside, surprisingly, it was neat and tidy. I called her name as I opened the door and received no response. It was eerily quiet except for the low hum of the oxygen concentrator. I walked slowly through a darkened living room, allowing my eyes to adjust to the light. Again, I called her name, hoping not to be shot as an intruder.

Many home care patients either leave their doors unlocked or have a key hidden by the door, and even though they know who will be visiting, some are still surprised when we arrive. Unless you have worked for a significant time in the home care industry, you cannot wholly appreciate the dangerous situations in which we are placed. We do not have the option to pick and choose our patients, their living conditions, or their state of mind. They forget, as we all have had memory lapses at times, and age, disease, medications, stress, anxiety, etc, further diminish cognition. And any idiosyncratic behavior can be magnified.

As I was about to enter the hallway that stretched to the end of the mobile home, I turned the corner, and I could see Penny sitting on the side of her bed in a haze of cigarette smoke. Her nasal cannula was in her lap, and a full-lit cigarette was in her hand. I froze. I yelled at her to put out the cigarette. An image of the mobile home flashed in my mind, engulfing it in flames with a simple flicker from that cigarette, trapping both of us in this tinder box. I yelled again for her to put out the cigarette, but this time, she reached for her nasal cannula. "NO! THE CIGARETTE! Put the cigarettes out! Put the cigarette out! " I yelled, with all my commands leaving my mouth in rapid succession.

"I need an ashtray," came the response.

An ashtray? Are you kidding me? Use your fingers or put it out on the table. How did you put out the others? These thoughts jumbled up in my mind, though I could say nothing.

There were a good thirty feet between me and her, with only one exit, which was behind me, and I thought, "We are not dying this way, not today."

At this point, I had three immediate choices:

- Turn around, leaving the way I came in, and call the hospice team.

- Go to her and try to take the cigarette from her, possibly dropping it and releasing an ember.

- Take something to her to place the cigarette in.

Since her room was full of cigarette smoke and she held a full-length cigarette in her hand, to me, this meant that this was not her first cigarette of the day. She had managed so far not to burn the house to the ground. Knowing this gave me a slight calmness, though there was still this clear and present danger.

The oxygen was still flowing from the nasal cannula in her lap, penetrating the fibers of her clothes, carpet, and bedding. If she dropped the cigarette or ash fell from the lit end, it would immediately ignite whatever it came into contact with, causing a fire that would spread faster than anyone could control or be saved from.

The hallway seemed to get longer with every millisecond. I did not want to continue down it, but I knew I could not leave. It was just one of those days I wished I had stayed in bed. However, I was already committed to this situation.

Noticing I was also standing adjacent to the kitchen and kitchen sink, I grabbed a cup from the sink and filled it with water. I told Penny I was bringing a cup of water for her to put her cigarette in. The water from the faucet seemed to move in slow motion as I steadied the cup just enough to fill it a quarter full. I could throw the water on whatever caught fire as a backup plan. However, depending on the material, it could spread a fire.

I took a deep breath, more like a sigh of resignation, and started down the hall. As I approached Penny, I could see her hand shaking, but so was mine. I'm not going to lie; I did not want to be in that situation and was a little scared. With every step I took, I could feel the hallway walls close in on me as if I were walking into a dark, abandoned mine shaft.

I needed just a few more steps to reach her. At that moment, she lifted the cigarette to her lips to take another puff. "No! In the cup!" I picked up my pace towards her. But she was determined to have that last puff, and so she did. Then she extended her arm towards me and unceremoniously plopped the cigarette into the cup.

Really? Was it that easy? There were no fireworks, I did not trip, and nothing caught on fire. My adrenaline was at a ten, and Penny, well, Penny, was utterly unaware of my end-of-the-world gloom and doom. She sat there as if she did not have a care in the world. It was then that I noticed her pupils were pinpoint. My head pivoted to her bedside table, and I saw the liquid morphine sulfate bottle alongside a few filled syringes and about six empty ones.

Are you serious? Let's review: Basically, a bed-bound patient who lives alone in a mobile home, has oxygen and is ventilator dependent, smokes, and is given a bottle filled with a mind-numbing narcotic to use as needed. Who puts a patient in this situation? Now I was angry.

After settling Penny, I excused myself to go outside and call the hospice home team. With the adrenaline still pumping through my veins, I could not dial the number fast enough to reach the clinical manager for that team.

After explaining the situation to the manager, her reply was: "She wasn't supposed to go home; the doctor ordered her to go to the hospice home."

"Then why is she home?" I was annoyed that I even had to ask that question.

"The admission nurse messed up and sent her home."

"You're blaming the admission nurse as to why this patient is alone, at home, medicated, and smoking."

"We had her sign a smoking waiver."

"A smoking wavier? A waiver that protects the company from liability but not the patient from the situation in which we have placed her?"

"Like I said, the admission nurse messed up, and she ended up at home."

"You have a doctor's order for her to be in a hospice home, but you leave her at home. I suggest you get a nurse out here as soon as possible to evaluate this situation and notify the physician of the patient's location."

I was angry. They don't care. To them, it's just a number on a data collection spreadsheet.

As I ended the call, the neighbor primarily caring for Penny arrived. I expressed my concerns and asked that he remove the cigarettes and lighter from Penny's room until the nurse arrived. He told me that he had already called the hospice office to tell them what was happening and to see if she could go to the hospice home. He was told a social worker would need to evaluate the patient to qualify for the hospice house. Hopefully, a different social worker would prefer to assess patients in person rather than over the phone.

Penny would be transported that day to the hospice home where, if she chose, she could be safely supervised to smoke on the patio. She passed away at that hospice home about three weeks later.

It would make for an interesting report/book to survey the fire departments in a given region for a specific period, say five to ten years, where hospice services were in place, noting which homes were involved, under what circumstances the fire occurred, living conditions/arrangements, and whether oxygen and/or medications played a role in the fire.

## Mercy Killing?

Not only does hospice play a role in the deaths of adults, but imagine a child—a child whose parents were actively discontinuing life support for their child who had Locked-in-Syndrome (LIS). With LIS, you can feel pain, hunger, loneliness, and fear but can't react to those sensations. You are aware of your surroundings, but you can't communicate your feelings or desires. Nothing in your body works except vertical eye movement and the ability to blink. This meant that the child was aware of what was happening but could not express himself.

The parents wanted him to die, so they were turning the respiratory rate on his ventilator down by two breaths per minute every ten minutes. Slow-motion suffocation. Can you imagine being dependent on a machine to breathe for you and slowly having those breaths taken away? You are receiving 12 breaths this minute, then only 10. And in a few minutes, you get only eight breaths. Then, 6. Your heart rate is 150, and you can feel the urge and sensation to breathe more, but you cannot. As your body begins to ache from the lack of oxygen and the panic feeling of being suffocated, you are now only given four breaths and no medication to ease his suffering.

According to a "leadership" manager, the hospice doctor who approved and told the parents what to do was on vacation in another town 60 miles away, probably sipping a margarita on a beach.

This child suffered a horrific murder at the hands of his parents, aided by an absentee doctor and covered up by a killing organization.

The wrong discharge

The wrong patient

The wrong equipment

The wrong medication

The wrong dose

The unnoticed death

The wrong time

The lack of staff

The forged signature

The wrong place

This list could go on and on....

Someone could argue that these items could be just "one-offs." Still, when you work in this environment, and you see daily the neglect, the patient complaints, the lack of concern from leadership, the policy changes that only benefit the organization, the staffing cutbacks, the lay-offs, positions posted only never to be filled (which serves to show they are "trying" to fill positions by not trying), the staff members who speak up and are terminated, no it is not "one-offs" - it is a systematic approach to maximize profits and deny required and mandated services.

This is further demonstrated by the leadership.

## Leadership? What Leadership?

Standing at the end of a long conference table, she looked to the person to her left and asked that they start the introductions. We had all been gathered to hear about, and more importantly, participate in, the yearly employee "giving" campaign.

At the table, the introductions went around the table, which included a couple of respiratory therapists, physicians, a nurse practitioner, and a speech therapist, then back to her, at which point she said, "Well, I'm your boss." The physician sitting next to me nearly choked on his water.

We will call her "Babbs". She was an EMT who had previously worked as a transport coordinator for the organization. My understanding is that she was given this management position as a favor and that the human resource department knew she did not qualify for the position, but we will get to that a little later.

The employee giving campaign, created by the organization's leadership, had a two-pronged approach. First, it was and continues to be a ruse for the organization to milk its employees for money and, second, more importantly, to deceive its community donors about true employee involvement through the manipulation of facts.

Employees are gathered by their manager for a meeting, usually in small groups, to watch a video presentation about the organization's "merits" and "good deeds". This presentation usually involves numerous employees performing various duties; all staged for the sake of filming the presentation.

The last one I viewed had just about every C-suite person in it. As I watched the film, I thought, "What a waste of time and money." Instead of the CEO and the other C-suite personnel spending their day frolicking in front of a camera playing James Bond or some superhero, they could just as easily donate one day's pay. But that wasn't the goal.

Babbs was so desperate to make a name for herself and to prove that she deserved the position she was given that during the giving campaign events, she would include a $5 bill in our envelopes.

Her instructions to us were that we could leave the $5 in the envelope and sign the form as a one-time donation, or we could take the money to buy lunch and fill out the form for a payroll deduction. She wanted 100% participation. With a participation rate of 100%, she would be highlighted in the monthly newsletter and receive kudos from leadership.

Following the presentation, the presenter would further note the importance of "giving back" to the organization and stress that each employee is expected to give a "donation." The leadership is expecting 90% overall participation, and the manager is hoping to have 100% participation. No pressure.

Then, each employee is given an envelope with their name printed on the outside. A preprinted form is contained within the envelope and divided into three sections. The top section includes the employee's personal information, such as name, department, etc. Another section on the form is a place for the employee to choose which part of the organization their donation should be directed to. Then, finally, how much money does the employee want to "give" to the organization, and in what form, and how often? Coercion comes to mind. Yes, it is that blatant.

However, gaining money back from the employee isn't the primary goal either. The goal comes from misrepresenting the facts of "employee participation" to the community donors. The organization has a whole department dedicated just to community donors. That's where the money lies. Donating to a hospice organization can help a community's deep pockets sleep better at night while also providing a nice tax write-off at the end of the year.

When an organization can show potential community money donors how active the employees are in giving back to the company, the train of thought is this: "If our employees give and believe in what we do, then you can as well."

The statistic of 90% employee involvement can speak volumes if it is accurate. Community donors are fleeced by deceptive statements and facts. Would these potential donors be so willing to give their money if they knew the employee backing was not as stated or presented, and that employees are pressured into donating or even being bribed to do so?

However, that could be her leadership style. However, during her tenure, Babbs created chaos all around her.

She would be on complex conference calls where the clinical staff discussed a patient with complex needs, and she would add her quarter's worth of no-nonsense. She would triage respiratory calls as if she were a therapist and even lead the nurses into thinking she was a therapist without correcting them.

One evening, I received a call from a hospice nurse stating she was calling as a follow-up from a previous call with a therapist. As this nurse detailed the last call with what instructions she received from "the other therapist" and what actions were taken, none of what she said made any sense. It made sense that what the nurse did would change the patient's status. Unfortunately, it was a negative change. At that point, I was suspicious whether the nurse had spoken to a therapist. Although the nurse had gotten half of the 'instructions' correct, they were applied in the wrong situation.

I could not imagine any of our therapists giving such instructions. So I asked her, "Who did you say you spoke to earlier?" "The other therapist, Babbs." Ahh, yes, so that would explain it.

It was a similar situation when I emailed the hospice team about a patient in service who was on a ventilator. The team physician wanted to know the difference between BiPAP and ventilator settings per the company policy. My explanation included the difference between the two modes of ventilation and why this patient needed one mode over the other.

A few weeks later, I was sent an email thread to get the back story on a patient coming into service. As I read the discussion, I came across a part of an email that was very familiar. It read exactly as I would write it. In fact, it was what I wrote about another patient, word for word.

Babbs had copied a paragraph I wrote about a patient and pasted it in an email to the hospice team about a different patient. She was making it seem as though she knew more than she did. The problem was that although the information was correct, it was not accurate when applied to this second patient. It would be contraindicated and potentially harmful.

Besides practicing respiratory therapy without a license, the worst part was that she didn't even know what she was talking about. I felt as though I was constantly in clean-up mode. Another therapist and I would comment that if she spent as much time doing the stuff she was supposed to be doing rather than trying to be an RT, our payroll would be correct, policies would be typed, or a hundred other things that she should have been doing but was not.

An example would be when one of our therapists gave up her full-time position with hospice. This therapist chose only to work as needed. This change in employment status necessitated a termination of employment and a rehire as a pool or per diem employee. Babbs did half the job. She terminated the employee in the system from her full-time position but neglected to submit the proper documents to the Human Resources department so the therapist could have a per diem position.

So, in essence, Babbs terminated an employee and failed to rehire her in another position. The problem? Babbs continued to schedule this therapist to work for hospice as a therapist for another six to eight weeks. And the therapist worked, thinking she was an employee, but she wasn't. The therapist continued to receive pay during this time because Babbs was manually entering payroll information, thinking there was something wrong with the system. This system allowed payments to a non-employee.

How many others outside the organization received payments without accountability, and for what? Perhaps patient referral kickbacks? Crazy, I know, but true.

We had another therapist who worked part-time during the day for hospice and worked at night for a local hospital. Unbeknownst to the other staff members, at night, when this therapist was on-call for hospice but at her hospital job, Babbs would answer the hospice therapist's on-call calls. She would triage calls, answer questions, and give instructions and recommendations as if she were the therapist.

Another time, she even directed a new hire therapist to see a patient in a facility who was pending discharge rather than visit a patient who was in respiratory distress on his ventilator at home. Why? Because the admission is more important than the safety of the patient.

You don't need to be a therapist to know that a stable patient in a controlled environment (hospital) can wait and that an unstable patient in an uncontrolled environment (home) would need to be seen first. Every reader of this book will get that answer right.

I don't even want to guess how she 'helped' the pediatric physician of whom she was the "boss," which may explain the previous 'Mercy Killing' story.

Over the last two years of my employment with hospice, Babbs and I were always at odds. As the senior therapist, I was put in the position of cleaning up her mess of clinical issues. This cleanup included correcting the medical recommendations she gave the nurses and physicians, instructions she gave other therapists, information on ventilators to our outside vendors, applying corporate clinical policy correctly, educating the nurses and physicians regarding equipment/application, and the list goes on.

She was trying to work as a therapist. However, her position was similar to that of an administrative assistant. It was a non-clinical position, like human resource personnel. She did not possess the educational level, the credentials, or the state license to do anything clinical, but that did not stop her from trying to impersonate a licensed therapist.

I tried for months to push her back into her lane, which was scheduling, payroll, etc., not clinical. All to no avail. Whenever she and I met to discuss these ongoing issues, she would say, "I know, I know," meaning she knew what she was doing and needed to stop. But things did not change.

Finally, it came to the point that I filed a complaint with my medical director and Human Resources. And what did that accomplish? Nothing. Yes, we met, and yes, they listened, said they would "look" into it, and agreed that she should not be involved in any clinical issues. But did anything change? Since the administration failed to take any necessary steps to remove Babbs from interfering with clinical issues, it encouraged her to go further.

For example, when I contacted the manufacturer of a specialty nebulizer, knowing that some of our patients would benefit from one, I asked them to send me some samples that I could present to our medical director and the other therapists. The box arrived at the corporate office, where Babbs took it to the chief clinical officer without notifying me of their arrival.

Babbs' way of getting back at me was to take this box of EZ-PAPs sent from the manufacturer and deposit them with the Chief Clinical Officer without an explanation. And that is where they sat, pushed into a forgotten corner, while patients could have benefited from such a device. Her vengefulness was not impacting me, but it was hindering the care of our patients.

Finally, one of my fellow therapists, who was at the corporate office every week or so, noticed this box of nebulizers in the office and retrieved it from the office corner. We could finally finalize the process of using these devices for the benefit of our patients, although it was too late for the specific patients I had in mind when I originally asked for them from the manufacturer.

At this point, I'm sure you are asking if she was genuinely interfering with clinical issues and she was not credentialed to do so; surely the administration would have removed her or reprimanded her. In hindsight, I can see how Babbs was the administration's foil. They used her as a buffer to carry out their agenda. They knew what she was doing, and they wanted it that way. She was doing their dirty work. She was too naive to know better or too ambitious to care. Either way, it worked out for the leadership of the organization.

She would later be terminated after the company had to pay employees their back pay for time worked off the clock over three years. We were pushed hard to finish everything while being told there was no overtime. At several meetings, she would brag that "all my staff" worked off the clock. She considered that a sign of devotion to her, not the job. While I appreciate that the organization took action to pay us for our off-the-clock work hours, it was too easy to get our back pay. Two questions from them: how many hours and for how long? They knew all along.

How many others do they owe for working hours off the clock who are afraid to speak up for fear of losing their job?

One therapist stated they got off easy with the back pay, which I agreed.

## Let's Talk Oxygen

Is the air we breathe and the water we drink all the same? The environment has been under attack since the Industrial Age, and the quality of these vital necessities will only continue to decline.

Oxygen is contained within the air around us. It allows us to live. It is an odorless, colorless gas that makes up about 21% of the Earth's atmosphere. We need this precious gas to sustain us physically. Still, for many, it can be a source of never-ending anxiety.

If you require oxygen in the hospital upon discharge, are you suddenly cured to the point where you no longer need it? You may need 10 liters of oxygen in the hospital. However, you have a 5-liter oxygen concentrator already at home, so you must be good to go home, right? Wrong.

Not all oxygen is the same. There are two ways to supply medical oxygen, which are very different.

Stationary oxygen concentrators

First, the majority of oxygen provided in the home will be supplied by a machine called an oxygen concentrator. It is about the size of a medium piece of luggage, has wheels, and is heavy. The oxygen concentrator runs off of electrical power, which plugs into the wall outlet with no backup battery.

There are two main parts of an oxygen concentrator: the compressor and the sieve bed. As the oxygen concentrator pulls room air into the unit, the compressor compresses all the air, and the sieve beds are filters that remove the nitrogen from the air. When the nitrogen is removed, the oxygen is left.

There are inherent problems with oxygen concentrators, such as:

-The oxygen produced is a warm, dry gas. It is recommended that an external water bubble humidifier be used for any flow rate greater than 4 LPM. Although, since the water bubble humidifier is made of cheap plastic and may not be easily accessible, many times the adaptor is mis-threaded, allowing oxygen to leak out around the connector. This oxygen leak goes back into the room and not to the patient.

-The lack of adequate maintenance of the sieve beds. The sieve beds contain zeolite that separates nitrogen from the oxygen in the air. The container of Zeolite pellets is either a replaceable cartridge or a refillable bed. It should be changed according to manufacturer guidelines for each make and model.

-Improper disinfecting and cleaning. Depending on the specific oxygen concentrator, it may have intake filters such as a grey reusable filter, an internal HEPA filter, an output bacterial filter, or none of these. These filters, or lack thereof, will impact the pressure output flow. Also, little creatures like the warm, dark environment will travel within the concentrator, staying within and traveling from patient home to patient home.

-The need for backup oxygen tanks. Since the oxygen concentrator needs electricity to operate, oxygen tanks are left in the home as a backup in the event of an electrical power loss. These tanks are heavy, require a regulator, and are a safety concern if not stored properly.

Additionally, the average 5-liter flow max concentrator has an average FiO2* of 86-90% and will cost the homeowner an average of $40-$60 per month of electrical usage. The 10-liter flow max concentrators are similar in FiO2*, and the average electric cost is higher. Also, the oxygen concentrator produces heat, so to further add to the electric cost of operating it, there is the extra electrical use to cool the home with the A/C. *FiO2-fraction of inspired oxygen

Side Note: A bedside fan or stick floor fan directed at the patient's face may help lessen the air hunger sensation as the air brushes the cheeks and forehead. It's not the same as an overhead fan's usage.

## Liquid Oxygen

The other type of oxygen is liquid oxygen, in semi-portable canisters. These canisters are similar in shape and size to a small water heater for home use. The liquid is converted to gas through a system of copper tubing. Liquid oxygen is 99.9% pure. A larger commercial system of bulk liquid oxygen is used to fill portable oxygen tanks.

Usually, a vendor specializing in this type of oxygen will set up two or three canisters in a home. These canisters can be linked together for a higher overall oxygen flow rate. Each canister's flow rate can be individually adjusted for up to 10 liters per minute. Some canisters have specialty regulators to allow a flow of 15 liters per minute (LPM). However, the most commonly used regulator is a 10 L and is usually used at 8 LPM to decrease the possibility of it becoming frozen.

Liquid oxygen is expensive, and most hospices do not offer it. However, there are some diseases that liquid oxygen best serves, such as Interstitial Lung Disease, like Pulmonary Fibrosis, or those that are sensitive to oxygen and can "feel" the difference.

## Brandon

One such patient, Brandon, was a young man in his 40s dying of lung cancer. I had visited him several times over the last couple of months of his life. Occasionally, he would mention that when he felt short of breath, he would use the oxygen from his portable oxygen tank (the green cylinder you've probably seen in a hospital). They are about three feet high and housed in a little cart with two wheels. I would tell him to use whatever he wanted. Over the months, his oxygen tank collection grew from one to about ten tanks—the tanks becoming his security blanket.

His health was declining rapidly, and he grew more dependent on the tank oxygen than on using his concentrator for oxygen. He could feel the difference between the two different types of oxygen, even though every nurse who visited him would insist that there was no difference. "Oxygen is oxygen," they would say over and over again. Surprisingly, even most physicians think there is no difference.

My last visit was mid-morning, about 10ish. I arrived to see an unfamiliar face who answered the door. I introduced myself, and in turn, this person explained that they were the neighbors who were asked to sit with Brandon this morning while his wife had to go to work. Brandon's wife had expressed concern to them the prior night, and they offered to stay with him. His wife had seen his ups and downs over the last couple of weeks, so while she was concerned, she also thought he would bounce back.

I entered the home to find Brandon sitting in his favorite reclining chair. Usually, he would be slightly reclined, but now he is sitting straight upright. As I approached him, his eyes flickered open, and he smiled briefly, then closed. He was wearing his nasal cannula and an additional oxygen mask attached to separate oxygen tanks.

He was doing his best to remain still, but the anxiety would break through, and he would shift in his chair. He asked me for more oxygen. I told him he was already on as much as possible. He then stated that he needed more tanks. I checked his tanks; he had about three full tanks plus his 10-liter concentrator. I asked him if I could change one of the oxygen devices to the concentrator. At that question, he became agitated, stating "that oxygen does not work."

"Please." Came the plea of a dying man. Looking at him, I knew that the tanks that would be delivered would last longer than he would. But that did not matter. What mattered was that it would give him some solace.

I asked the neighbors sitting with Brandon what medications he had been given. They showed me the medication list and the times they were last given. All the medication had been given as ordered, and I could see that the team nurse had been out about an hour earlier and increased his morphine and Xanax. I also inquired when the wife would be back - "shortly after five."

I told Brandon I would step outside, make a few phone calls, and be right back in.

I first called the team nurse to inquire if she had requested a nurse in the home from the continuous care team.

"Yes, but no one is available. Maybe at 8 pm, they will have someone available."

"He will be dead and cold by then. Why do we promise services that we cannot fulfill?"

"I know. Did you tell the neighbors to call the wife home?"

"No, not yet." How can people not take ownership of a situation and do the right thing? Does it really take much more effort to do one or two more things to help a patient other than just placing a check in a box on a checklist? "Would you please continue to work to get a nurse to the bedside?"

"Sure"

I then called the warehouse to ask for additional oxygen tanks to be delivered. The warehouse secretary, Kitty, answered the phone. Kitty was the type of employee who, if she didn't have to do it, she wouldn't, or if she could get someone else to do it, they did it. I gave her the patient's name and requested ten additional oxygen tanks delivered "as soon as possible, as in the next hour."

Kitty says, "He already has ten in the home and a concentrator; he doesn't need any more."

"He doesn't need any more," rang in my ears as if someone had slapped me upside the head. "He doesn't need any more." A secretary, sitting at a desk in an office, thinking about what she was going to have for lunch, is telling me, who is at the bedside of a dying man, "He doesn't need any more."

I spoke slowly and deliberately-"Kitty, get a driver over here with tanks within the next hour, or I'll come to the warehouse and bring them myself." I was furious.

"I'll have to talk to Bill" (Bill being the warehouse manager), and she hung up.

I went back into the home and stayed by the front door to ask the neighbor to call the wife for me to speak with.

After telling the wife about my assessment, I suggested she might want to come home. She asked if today was the day, and I thought so. She asked how long, and I said, "Probably a few hours, maybe through the night." This may sound like a strange conversation, so matter-of-factly, but the patient and wife have anticipated this day for months.

Another young man I had helped months earlier so eloquently put it into words: "We are not extending life; we are delaying death." And for Brandon, the delay was no more.

The neighbors standing close by were surprised by what I said to the wife. "You think he is going to die?" Was that a question? I looked at them and then looked at Brandon. I wanted to say, "Do you not see what I see?" Or, "Yes, this is what lingering death looks like," but all I could do was nod. "But he is still awake and talking," he said. Again, all I could do was nod. At that point, I knew they wanted more answers, but I was unconcerned with their questions; my focus was on Brandon.

I went to Brandon to make a few adjustments to his oxygen and to reposition him in his chair. As I sat beside him, he moved his hand towards me, and I placed his hand in mine. At that point, he just wanted to connect with someone he felt would know what was what. He was tired. His whole body was limp as he closed his eyes and seemed to be mentally at peace. However, his body betrayed that peacefulness with the exhausting effort to breathe. We sat in silence.

I would leave his side with a promise to get extra oxygen tanks to him within an hour. He nodded with the same knowing nod I gave the neighbors.

As I pulled up to the warehouse, the only parking space available was right outside Bill's office. As soon as my foot touched the inside of the building, I heard, "Michelle, I've sent those tanks," echo down the hall. That was Bill. He would calm my fire before it could get out of control. Bill was also a therapist and always prioritized the patient's care. He was one of the original therapists, an old-timer. He blazed the trail for the rest of us to follow. He gave me my first job in respiratory services while I was still in college at a small, family-owned hospital in Tampa. And then, thirty-odd years later, by chance, we would meet up, and he would hire me for a second time, this time for hospice. Bill was a smart man. He would retire from hospice, looking forward to spending time with his wife, kids, and grandkids at his home in the hills of Tennessee, only to lose his fight with cancer. Bill will be missed in the respiratory community.

I went straight to his office. As I entered his office, he immediately stated that the tanks I requested were already on their way. However, I did not cognitively hear him and immediately told him what I thought of the office staff and the lack of empathy the warehouse secretary displayed. Not only on this day, but this day was the final straw. Then Kitty appeared in the doorway and again stated: "That patient has ten tanks and a concentrator. He doesn't need any more tanks." I can not tell you how much that was wrong to say to me, again, at that moment.

Let me clarify that there have been only three times in my career that I have pulled the "I'm the Therapist" card in the thirty years I have worked in healthcare. Once was twenty-odd years ago with a physician fresh out of school and twice with hospice. The other was with my EMS tech/pseudo manager, which was discussed earlier.

"Kitty, YOU are the secretary. I'm the therapist. Do not tell me what my patients do or do not need. If I tell you they need something, it is NOT your place to question me or my judgment."

This is the type of disconnect that is so prevalent in the healthcare system. We have frontline clinicians dealing face-to-face with death, dying, and disease daily. Then we have office staff who lack empathy because their day is filled with numbers, quotas, and inventory. What difference does it make if ten oxygen tanks are in a warehouse collecting dust or placed in a patient's home to calm the patient? Other than the thirty minutes it would take the driver, round trip, to make that delivery. Oh, and the effort of the secretary to enter a delivery ticket.

These are simple services that should and could be provided to patients. What may look insignificant to the non-clinician and can be easily dismissed as such really does have a huge impact. It just takes someone to care enough to take ownership of the situation and provide a layer of compassion and dignity to those we serve.

Brandon passed away around 7 pm that night.

## A Son's Mom

People are funny. Not in a laugh-out-loud way but in the customs that we continue with our pleasantries when we meet someone for the first time. There is the usual "Are you married?" and "How many kids do you have?" Those two questions always go hand in hand. The assumption is that if you are married, you must have kids.

The same can be said when it comes to the career part. So, as soon as I say hospice, I can see the physical uneasiness manifest itself with the shifting of the feet, the lowering of the head, and the avoidance of eye contact. "Oh, you work for hospice." "I could never do that type of work," as if some taboo subject had reared its head. And then there is the look of pity or surprise or a combination of both, like when you work with dying or dead people. Yes, I do. And I hate to tell anyone something they may not know, but you will die, too. We all will at some point, so you might as well plan and prepare for it.

According to the team nurse's email, Bobby was 47 years old with lung cancer. Over the last several days, the nurse has increased his oxygen from 4 liters per minute (LPM) to 6 LPM per nasal cannula. That in itself does not sound too alarming.

I made arrangements with the family to be at his home around noon that Thursday. I pulled up to a light yellow home with white shutters that had the appearance of an old plantation home. It had a wrap-around porch and was sitting on a couple of acres of land shaded by massive oak trees.

As I pulled into the driveway, I was greeted at my car door by an elderly gentleman, I'd say, who was in his late 60s or early 70s, followed by a golden retriever. The gentleman was solemn, not saying much, which starkly contrasted to the golden retriever, who was overjoyed at the newcomer. The gentleman pointed out a shady spot next to the house for me to park, and he told me to "just go on in," motioning toward the front door area. He thanked me, and then the two were off, retreating to the backyard.

Upon stepping onto the front porch, a woman of similar age opened the door. "Thank goodness you are here." She introduced herself as the aunt, stating her sister was there with her nephew. As she anxiously led me down a hallway, my thoughts were, "OK, he's only on 6 LPM via nasal cannula. If you all cannot handle it now, what are you going to do when he's dying?"

Rounding the corner into his room, a young man was sitting straight up in his bed. Every bone in his body was visible as the skin was stretched like a leather wrap. Not an extra ounce of fat or muscle. He sat up high in the bed, his chest heaving with each breath. The veins in his neck pulsated. He was restless, moving about in the bed. The more he moved, the worse his breathing became. I asked him a few questions to gauge his awareness. He moaned in pain and said barely verbal partial words. He had all the signs of terminal agitation and was transitioning into the actively dying stage.

I was not prepared for this scenario. Although when we enter a home, we never know what we will find, we have an idea that a patient on low-flow oxygen and a patient at death's door are two different things and have completely different mindsets. I had to switch gears quickly.

His mom and aunt were at the bedside, waiting to help their loved one, but unsure as to what to do. I asked if they had any morphine and when was the last time it was given.

It was due to be given an hour ago. I suggested they give him a small dose now. It was liquid morphine. This type of morphine is drawn up in a syringe and given sublingually (under the tongue). It is very fast-acting. Liquid morphine, better known by its brand name, Roxanol, really is an end-of-life best friend in small doses.

As the aunt retrieved the bottle, the mom asked how much to give. My answer: how much is ordered? As the mom gave the morphine, I asked the aunt for the hospice binder. I wanted to see what his code status was without actually having to ask. As I flipped through the binder, I saw the yellow DNRO form. However, it was not completed. At this point, this gentleman was still a full code. If something was to happen, like what was happening, I was obligated to call 911 for him to be resuscitated.

Outside in the hallway, I explained this to his mom since, although he was not a DNRO, he did have in place a properly executed proxy document that would allow his mom to make decisions on his behalf, whether or not he had the mental capacity to do so on his own.

She seemed taken aback by this as if she was not expecting him to die. Her look concerned me as if realizing the situation was not hitting home. She asked, "What does that mean? What will they do if you call 911?" I told her what happened during the resuscitation process, and her response to me was, "You think he is dying? Now? How long do you think he has?"

Like so many other families, are they not seeing what I see? Is their hope of recovery or the hope of having just one more day blinding them to the reality in front of them?

I told her that I believed he had a few hours to a day. It was a Thursday early afternoon. I didn't think he would even make it through to the next day. She said her other sons were arriving the following Monday, four days away. She asked if they should come earlier. All I could do was nod yes. My first thought was that they wouldn't make it in time, but I couldn't say that to a mother standing in front of me, her dying son just feet away. His body was tired and worn out. He was dying and would be dead in a matter of hours.

The strange thing about working in this environment is that, although it is not for us to know when and where death will happen, one becomes very good at predicting death or recognizing its signs. And it's not any particular sequence of signs but more of a feeling. Over the years of seeing patients at the end stages of life, one becomes acutely aware if one pays attention.

Too many times, DNRO decisions are not made in advance. People wait. Waiting for what I don't know. If you have cancer throughout your body and begin to have a multi-organ shutdown, it's pretty much a done deal. Why force your loved one to make that decision? It's your life. Choose it. And obviously, this young man wanted to choose life. However, life was not a choice for him. Only more pain and agony. It was a very, very sad situation.

The mom instructed 911 not to be called, saying she just wanted him to be comfortable. I immediately called the attending physician to notify him of the situation. He agreed with the DNRO and requested that a continuous care nurse be sent to the home. When a continuous care nurse is in the home, they take over the administration of medications, allowing the family members to be a loving family and grieve rather than be caretakers. It takes away the burden. I informed the family that a team nurse was on the way. The mom began to cry. She stated that she loves her son very much and does not want to be left alone with him if he dies. She was still thinking in terms of "if," not "when."

I waited for the team nurse to arrive and gave her an update on the preceding events. She gave him some more sedation to ease the agitation and then proceeded to complete the needed DNRO documents. I asked the nurse to call for a chaplain, but the chaplain was on "vacation." I told her of the mom's request not to be left alone. The nurse said she would stay.

The following day, I checked the computer to see his status. He passed away at around midnight. The nurse said she would stay and left the house shortly after I left. She left the mom alone to care for, medicate, and grieve for her son. Chances are the nurse gave the young man a nice, healthy nursing dose of morphine to send him into a relaxing slumber until his death.

What could have been more important than staying with a dying patient, a person, a son? Nothing. Nothing could be more important unless you are in hospice. I'm not even going to say it.

It still amazes me the lack of empathy and compassion that healthcare clinicians display.

If the family was afraid to give any morphine during the transitioning phase, God helped that young man when he was in the actively dying stage. I can only hope that he had given up the fight by then. Otherwise, without proper medication for symptom management, he would have died a horrible death, and his poor mom would have been forced to watch.

What's the point of hospice if we are not there during the most critical time? Of course, for hospices, dying is not the critical time.

And for other patients, it's not hospice to fear...

## Don't Ask, Don't Tell

Healthcare providers are not immune to the unexplainable questions that linger long after the event. We may have doubts about the facts, and we question those doubts. Is it what we think it is, or is it something completely different?

I arrived at an ill-kept home and set off the road amongst a cluster of trees. I gingerly stepped through the overgrown grass to reach the wooden porch. I watched my footing as I walked up the mold-covered steps and over the missing and warped wooden boards.

A man in his fifties answered the door, clearly looking like he had had a rough life. I stepped into the trailer to the stench of old and new cigarette smoke mixed with a dash of old urine. Just to the left of the door was a hospital bed. It had been positioned so the back of the head of the bed was closest to the door. The elderly lady confined to the bed could not see who entered or exited the home. The bedside commode was just adjacent to the bed, filled with the day's activities. Her half-eaten sandwich was on her bedside table.

Mrs. Taylor, in bed, called out, "Johnny, who is it? Johnny, Johnny". A beautiful, bright smile came to Mrs. Taylor's face as I walked around the side of the bed to introduce myself. She reached her hand towards mine. Just as I was about to speak to her, I could "feel" the presence of someone standing behind me.

Right behind me, like a warm breath on my neck. I quickly turned to see another man standing within inches of my face. He startled me to the point where I nearly fell backward into the patient's bed.

He just stood there, void of any emotion. "Don't you be afraid. That's my brother, Joseph," said the man who greeted me at the door, "Joseph, get out of the lady's way." Joseph backed up a few steps but just stood there looking at me with an emptiness in his eyes. "He doesn't mean any harm; he's just a little slow." I started to turn back to Mrs. Taylor. However, an odd feeling was beginning to set in, and I paused. I moved to the bottom of the bed to speak with the patient while seeing, I mean, including the two brothers.

Usually, when I go into questionable situations or homes, I text or send my location to a co-worker or, at times, my brother. Although, really, what good would that do other than to give them a place to start looking for my cold, dead body? I've even had two patients pull a gun on me, but that's a story for another time.

As I spoke to the patient, she was quite pleasant, alert, and well aware of her surroundings. As the patient and I were discussing her medications and oxygen usage, her son, Johnny, interrupted us and asked about her morphine. Specifically, how much morphine could she take?

Morphine had been administered to make her breathing easier and more comfortable. I responded to Johnny by saying that she could take the amount prescribed on the medication label.

She had ordered two types of morphine. One was a slow-release tablet, and the other was liquid. The slow release was just as the name implies; the pill slowly dissolved, releasing the medication into the body over several hours. The liquid morphine, placed under the tongue, was to be used for any breakthrough shortness of breath or pain.

Both of these medications were on her bedside table. I read the instructions from the label to the patient and her sons. I noticed on the label that the prescription was two weeks old. I asked if she had been taking the medications as prescribed and if she thought they were helping her. Yes, to both. The son again asked, but this time, he asked how much would be too much.

Now, this in itself is not an unusual question. Many patients are afraid to take medications that they have not taken in the past, especially medications such as morphine, considering the negative connotation society has placed on its use.

I answered the question with a question, "Has your Mom used the medications as ordered over the last two weeks without any problems?"

"Of course."

"Then, the dose that is ordered is fine. Just stick to how it is ordered. If you have any questions about changing the amount or switching to a different medication, please speak to your nurse or doctor when they visit. Or you can always call the office and speak to your team's clinical manager."

I then turned to the patient, asking if she was alright taking her medications, "Yes," and if she was having any problems, "No."

I finished my visit with education on oxygen safety, not smoking in the home, and reviewing the office and after-hours phone numbers. As I was about to leave, the patient reached out her hand to grab mine, asking when I would be out again. I told her I would be out in about a week. Her face drooped slightly, which is not unusual given that these patients are happy to see and speak to anyone who can connect them to the outside world.

As I left this patient's home, I thought I should call the nurse and tell her I had completed my visit, but it was late, after hours, and it could wait until the morning.

It was about mid-morning when I could finally email the team nurse regarding my visit with Mrs. Taylor. I had to open her chart to find the names of the team manager and the attending physician and include them in a copy of the email. This is something I typically do. However, what was unexpected was that when I opened Mrs. Taylor's chart, it recorded her as deceased.

Is he gone? She was eating, drinking, and talking yesterday... now dead? Of course, there is the chance that she died in her sleep from a heart attack, and yes, it is hospice; the patients do die, but as I read the word "deceased," my mind became a vortex of thoughts reliving my entire time in that home: the questions, the sons, the look on her face when I left.

I immediately picked up my cell phone and called the team nurse. As the nurse answered her phone, I didn't even take the time for the usual phone pleasantries; I wanted an answer, and I wanted it now. What happened to Mrs. Taylor? Her chart shows her as deceased. "

Of course, the nurse knew who was calling, although she was not expecting that question. Oh, I'm not sure. One of the sons called the after-hours service to say she had passed away. I then told her about my visit, the sons, and the questions. "Yeah, I think both the sons were a bit off," she responded.

Then I said something I thought I would never say and received a response that I thought I would never hear.

"Do you think they killed her?"

"It happens all the time," she said.

## Companions

Following my GPS, it directed me down a long dirt road lined with mobile homes, each placed on its patch of dirt. They appeared to be dilapidated with blue tarps on the roof, front doors covered with bedsheets, broken windows, windows covered with wood panels, and front steps made of concrete blocks. It was as if I had stumbled upon a mobile home graveyard.

However, there were obvious signs that these were still being used as homes by someone, like the single chair and table covered with fast food bags, beer bottles, and the occasional car. The road ended at a high wall of metal panels pieced together in no particular order, looking like something out of Madmax. Great, now comes the feat of turning around without getting stuck in the sand.

Finally, making my way to the correct road, which was one over; the homes were a little better kept, but only by a little. I found my destination by creeping my car along and trying to decipher the house numbers.

After knocking at the door, I stepped back a few steps to wait for the door to open. Nothing. I knocked again. This time, I heard footsteps, and a well-fed face appeared in the door's window. However, as fast as that face appeared, it disappeared. And still, I stood there listening to the stillness, with the occasional chirp of a bird in a nearby tree. The tranquility abruptly ended with the piercing scream of "What the F*** is someone here for?" came a female voice from within the home, followed by distant stomping, which grew louder until finally, the door swung open, revealing a robust figure who, without a word, turned and walked away.

With much hesitation, I slowly entered the home. It was an oversized mobile home. Running along the left side of the mobile home was a very spacious living room, completely void of any furniture. To the immediate right, in what would be a dining room, was a sofa facing a large flat-screen TV and a coffee table that held a dirty ashtray, cigarettes, and lighter.

"Hello? Mrs. Hilda?"

"She's right there," said the robust figure, pointing to a room behind my right side. I turned towards that doorway to see an elderly lady sitting on the side of her bed, probably all of 80 lbs soaking wet. Her frail body was contained within a stained nightgown. Her bed was a rumpled mess of sheets and blankets on which two little dogs, one curled up near the back of the bed and one standing as if on guard, also made it their bed.

I entered her room, which looked like a catch-all room with a mattress pushed up against one wall. With an embarrassed smile, Mrs. Hilda apologized for the daughter's abruptness, "She's not a morning person"—it was 2 pm. "That's quite alright. I'm not much of a morning person either," I responded, as now her daughter had also made her way into the room.

"No, it's not that; she never tells me when someone is coming over."

"Well, I forgot, darling."

"Then write it down."

"I try to."

After about a minute of this back and forth between mother and daughter, the odor of something burning, like burnt toast, was present in the air. The daughter's face froze for a second before she realized that something in the kitchen needed her attention. As she hastily left the room, she called back over her shoulder, "See, this is what happens."

After a few minutes of exchanging pleasantries with Mrs. Hilda, I started my assessment, noting that she was not using her oxygen. When I inquired about the oxygen usage, she said she didn't need it. The daughter then reappeared, stating that her mom does not use her oxygen because "she's afraid to use it because I smoke."

"As long as you smoke outside, there isn't a problem."

"I only smoke outside."

"No, you don't, baby," Mrs. Hilda said quietly.

"Well, if it's hot or raining, I cannot go outside. And you smoke, did you tell her that? "

I changed the subject, hoping to lower the tension by commenting on her cute little dogs. Well, that was the wrong subject.

"I hate those dogs, and that one does nothing but whine all day." The daughter's face was starting to turn red. "Even at night, he does nothing but whine." She was referring to the little one cuddled up towards the back of the bed. He was practically hairless, and what hair he did have left covered a scaly, flea-covered body and a fat belly. As he tried to scratch his ear, he would wince and give a little yelp. All the signs of a dog needing help.

Mrs. Hilda reached back and patted the little dog. "He needs to visit a vet, but I don't have the money."

"I don't know why you have to have dogs; cats are better. I have two around here somewhere. One is named Cujo. He's my favorite." Cujo? Isn't that the name of a fictional evil dog? Although, in this situation, it seemed fitting that the daughter would use that name for her pet. "When you're gone," the daughter continued, "I'm throwing them out the door." And she was not kidding. I believe she meant it. This time, I did not acknowledge the daughter; I focused on Ms. Hilda.

I finished visiting Mrs. Hilda by offering a chaplain and social worker. I also added that I do animal rescue, and if Mrs. Hilda needed someone to take the dogs and get them the care they needed, I would find them a good home.

As I left that home, I called the team and requested a social worker and chaplain to visit Mrs. Hilda. I told the team's clinical manager about my visit, and she was not surprised by the daughter's behavior.

Early the next week, I received a call from the social worker. She asked if I had offered to take Mrs. Hilda's dogs.

"Yes, I did."

"She asked if you would come and get him."

"Who is he?"

"The little one that cries."

"What about the other one?"

"She said she could not give that one up yet."

Additionally, I asked the social worker to meet me there to witness Mrs. Hilda freely surrendering her dog and making it clear that the dog would not be returning.

The drive to her home felt like an eternity, although it was only about 40 minutes. When I arrived, the social worker was talking with Mrs. Hilda, stating she did not have to give her dog up. Mrs.

Hilda said she could not provide what the dog needed and that it was in the best interest of the dog.

As I placed the towel around the dog and picked him up, he seemed to tense up and relax. He was old and tired. Mrs. Hilda cried and thanked me. I quickly made my exit.

I drove straight to Dr. Rivers' office, the veterinarian I use for my animals. I briefly gave him the scenario and asked him to do whatever he needed to help this little dog. He took the dog from me for X-rays. A few minutes later, he returned without the dog.

"I think he's roughly 15–16 years old, with no teeth." Dr. Rivers stated, "He has tumors in his abdomen, CHF with pulmonary edema, and he has several fractures along his spine." I couldn't even speak; the pain that the dog must have endured with each movement and me picking him up. "I'm going to go back and put him down," he finished. All I could do was nod my head. As he opened the door to leave, he turned to me and said, "No amount of money in the world is going to save that dog."

No, just $161 and a lot of tears driving home.

I know this is entirely off-topic. However, I would be remiss if I did not include a voice for the truly voiceless.

As passionate as I am about caring for others who are constantly under attack and fall prey to our healthcare system, their furry companions are also at risk.

Yes, I stopped for turtles in the road, moving them out of harm's way in the direction they were headed. I've taken home plenty of abandoned or unwanted pets.

An Angora rabbit, abandoned by a mom of two kids who left her husband. The rabbit was caged in a filthy, dust- and cobweb-covered small birdcage that was too small for the rabbit to turn around. The white hair, now grey from dirt, matted, and with mites, hung from an almost lifeless body to the vet and then to the farm.

A baby duck, about three months old, was kept in a five-gallon bucket on the front porch. The bucket is covered with a steel grate. A brick was at the bottom of the feces-covered bucket to hold the bucket in place and keep it from toppling over. Due to the bucket and brick size, the webbing on one foot of the duck could not lie flat, causing the webbing to be partially deformed. The owners stated it was given to them, and they were waiting for it to get a little older before releasing it.

How much older would it be without food and water and living in that filth? They relinquished it to me. My sister added the duck to her ever-growing animal rehab 'farm' where the chickens, dogs, cats, etc., all live harmoniously and play together.

Within weeks of the duck playing with the dogs in the kiddie pool and trying to be a chicken, its webbed feet flattened out, and it could walk normally. Although I don't think my sister intended to have such a collection, she does have a way with animals.

I have visited too many older adults without family or friends who have no one to take care of their beloved companions. The pet is thrown outside to fend for itself or taken to a shelter when they pass.

According to the American Society for the Prevention of Cruelty to Animals (ASPCA), approximately 6.5 million companion animals enter U.S. animal shelters annually.

> Be a hero, be a voice for the voiceless.
> Adopt a family member; don't buy a pet.

## If It Starts Off Badly

As I drove through different counties to visit my patients, my car had turned into a second home. My office was on wheels, where I would spend eight or more hours each day during the week. The passenger seat is my desk, where my purse, laptop, and lunch are arranged. Although the arrangements vary by the time of day, it's a lovely retreat. I can tune out the noise of the day with smooth jazz or give myself a headache listening to talk radio. Either way, it's my little cocoon on wheels.

I pulled into the assisted living facility parking lot and looked for a shady parking spot. I'm blinded by the sun's reflection on other cars, the pavement, and buildings. As I exited from my little cocoon, I shielded my eyes. I made my way to the assisted living facility's entrance. The doors open as I approach, and I walk into the cool entryway. I pause just inside the doors to let my eyes adjust. I look around to see I am alone in an ornately decorated foyer. Sitting areas on either side are decorated with dark wood furniture and beautiful wall artwork. The bookcases stuffed with novels are within reach of the high-back reading chairs and sofa. Fresh flowers were neatly arranged on the coffee table, and off to one side was a sizable self-serve coffee station complete with a lemonade dispenser with what looked like fresh ice and lemon slices floating within. There was even a little basket filled with single-serve cookies and snacks. "Nice," I thought to myself. It even smelled fresh and clean, not what I expected.

Just as I was about to walk down the hall, a bright-eyed, grin-from-ear-to-ear young woman appeared and, in a sing-song voice, asked if I needed assistance. I notice her eyes wander over to my ID badge. Her smile disappeared just as quickly as it had appeared. Her voice was now almost monotone. "Oh, just sign in; you know where you are going," and then she disappears behind a closed door. "Sign in where?" I thought. This was my first time visiting this facility. I again looked around and noticed a small desk behind me along the wall with a notebook. The cover contains a printed "Home Health" label. I opened the book to find alphabet-lettered dividers. I start with the letter from my company, but the page begins with a patient's name. Strangely, they have arranged this book by the patient's name. So I turn to the 'K,' and there is my patient. All the residents' names and room numbers are in this book. The page shows each visitor's time and day. A book kept right by the door?

After signing in, I made my way down the first hallway, passing by the "game" room on one side of the hall, which was empty, and the physical therapy room on the other side of the hall. Through the glass wall dividing the PT room from the hallway, I could see six wheelchairs lined up and filled with elderly patients. One patient sat looking as if he was in a daze. A couple of patients eagerly tried their best to lift the hand weights up and down, extending their arms above their heads. One sat quietly, watching the TV. Two others sitting next to each other were in a lively conversation, exchanging the facility's gossip. The last wheelchair was still occupied, even though the resident had managed to wiggle his butt to the edge of the seat and was nearly on the floor. I stepped towards the window to tap on it to get the attention of the attending therapist, sitting at a desk appearing to be charting. Still, I stopped short when I noticed the therapist jump from his chair and race toward the wiggle worm. Accidents avoided

The hall ended at an intersection, prompting me to check the wall map for directions to my intended destination. A short right, then a short left, and then a long hall to yet another turn down a hallway. The building did not look this big from the outside, and what started as bright and airy now seems to have become dimmer and confining.

As I approached the last corner, I faced what I had initially expected upon entering this building. The smells, the sights, and the sounds are unique to the enclosed living environment of those dependent on others for their care.

The medicinal odor combined with old urine is a familiar combination that only seems to happen in nursing homes and ALFs. The sight of wheelchair after wheelchair lined up along the wall with the same mix of patients I saw in the PT room. Only these patients were less 'alert' and, to add to the mix, there were a few patients who looked as though they had had a stroke, with one side of their body limp and drool running down their face. Others tried to move their wheelchairs by shuffling and pushing with their feet, with no luck because the wheels of the wheelchairs were locked or they were up against a wall. Try as they might, they were going nowhere.

And the gentleman who sat in the corner of the last hall. He looked a little younger than the others but still had a dazed look in his eyes. The bewildered look could be from a brain injury or medically induced by the nursing staff. He sat, wearing only a diaper, in an upright wheelchair, basically a tall back chair with wheels. It was fitted with a tray in front of him—a form of restraint—which confined him to the chair. As I passed him, three aides stood behind him, looking at his back with fascination and excitement on their faces. They were discussing the best way to pop that "big mother." I can only imagine their interest in a pimple on the patient's back.

And then the sounds of such a place: one patient's odd moaning, another calling out "nurse," and still others with a never-ending cry for help from "confused" patients. It is the kind of place that we all must think about and say to others, ' Don't let me end up here'. However, people do end up here. Were those the same wishes expressed by the people who are here now?

Finally, I found my way to her room.

Normally, when we transfer a patient home on special equipment or for extenuating circumstances, a nurse would do a home safety check before transferring the patient home. The safety check would include:

Verifying the home had electricity.
Running water.
A bed for the patient.
Sufficient workspace.
Perhaps a way into the home.

But, as with other nonproductive or non-billable activities, these little details did not matter anymore. And whether we agreed or not, we learned how to overcome any obstacle to achieve the goal. Our goal is to take care of the patient, as opposed to leadership's goal of increasing profits.

I entered Ms. Kab's room to find her in a bariatric bed, a wider version of a regular hospital bed that will accommodate larger body frames. In this particular case, the larger body frame was nearly 400 lbs.

Ms. Kab was dying from respiratory failure associated with COPD. She had been prescribed a BiPAP unit to use at night while she slept. However, the "at night" usage then became usage during the day. Then, as her disease state progressed, so did her need for use of the BiPAP. She was now using it every day, all day and night. She could not remove the BiPAP mask for more than a few minutes. She now wished to be taken home and withdrawn from the life support that the BiPAP had become.

I do not recall the exact circumstances surrounding her admission. However, I clearly remember arriving at her home. Her home is a tiny, framed cottage with a single door in the middle, preceded by a narrow walkway. Clearly, a home was built when people were not so tall or well-fed.

I stood at the back of the ambulance as Ms. Kab was readied for her final stretcher ride into the house. As I watched the paramedics, the hospice nurse stood next to me and asked: "How do you think we can get her into the home?" I just smiled, not knowing what she meant. I looked at the nurse, then at the front door, then at the stretcher, and back to the nurse. "Let's go look," I suggested. As we approached the door, I could see two issues.

The first issue was that the door was narrow. I mean really narrow, like way before ADA concerns. The second issue was the wall. A wall was just inside the doorway, barely three feet from the door. Once inside the door, one would turn right into the kitchen or left into the living room. Either way, a stretcher would not make that turn.

Awesome. This would have been an ideal situation to have that home safety inspection done before my arrival. Maybe there's a side door, "she whispered in my ear, not to concern the gathered family members.

We were back to square one once we noticed the fencing surrounding the backyard, blocking the side doors. As we turned to go back to the ambulance, one of the paramedics was right behind us, verbalizing the whole situation as we had just surveyed it. "Yes, that's correct," I answered.

"Well, we will just have to slide her in," he quipped.

Slide her in? Slide her? "Wait, what do you mean, 'slide her in'?"

"Oh, we do it all the time. It's no biggie. "His confidence almost convinced me.

I listened in horror as he detailed the situation to his partner. He planned to use a blanket underneath Ms. Kab and drag her over the step, through the door, around the wall, down the hall, and into the bedroom. Once in the bedroom, everyone available would help lift her into the bed. "Yes, I think that will work!" The nurse chirped.

"What? Do you agree with that plan? "I asked her.

"Sure, what choices do we have? Take her back to the ALF?" She answered.

The paramedics placed the stretcher as close to the door as possible, but it still seemed like a very long way away. This plan mortified me, even more so as the neighbors gathered in the yard. It was becoming a sideshow.

As the four of us huddled together to solidify the game plan, we asked the family to move all the furniture to one side of the living room, clear the hallway, and clear the bedroom. We would need a clear shot. Ms. Kab would not be able to take much stress, and there would be a short time she would be off the BiPAP.

The confident paramedic readied Ms. Kab by explaining the plan and assuring her that she would be wrapped up like a little papoose. Ms. Kab only nodded.

Then, the physician arrived. "No, you will not drag my patient on the ground and through the house."

And the nurse once again asked, "Take her back to the ALF?"

As promised, the paramedics constructed their little papoose and finished just as it started to rain. Perfect. All hesitation was gone now, as were the prying neighbors. Good.

Ms. Kab was pushed off the stretcher with one good heave and plopped on the concrete walk.

One paramedic by her head was pulling on the blanket, while the other was at her feet. They had hoped to slide her across the stoop and through the doorway, but the rough concrete had other ideas.

At least up to the doorway, we adjusted the slide board under Ms. Kab. At this point, we realized no one had adjusted for the body mass spread from Ms. Kab's lying on a solid surface. A good six inches of body flesh spilled out past the door frame on either side.

At this point, Ms. Kab was half in and half out of the front door. We now needed to get her completely through the door, turn left, and at least into the living room.

And to add to this, there was another problem. From the months of her lying in a bed, and due to her size, she was not flexible enough to pull her knees up, which means that, although we may be able to get her body through the doorway, how would we get her legs turned? She was taller than three feet, so once through the door, her head would touch the wall just beyond the door, and her legs and feet would still be outside.

And if that was not enough, the family stood watching. As you can imagine, emotions run very high during such situations. Not only do you have family members who get along with each other and genuinely care about the well-being of their loved ones, but you also get angry families that resolve their differences by physically fighting in the front yard following the withdrawal of life support from their loved ones. Yes, that has happened as well.

Families during these times are funny. Sometimes it's ha-ha funny, and sometimes it's downright scary funny. Unfortunately, we never know what will transpire until it happens and the police respond. Box of chocolates.

Most family issues during this difficult time are usually due to varying opinions on the right course of action to take. One child agrees with a DNR, while another wants everything done to save their parent. Or the new wife who signs the DNR on her husband against the acceptance of the stepchildren.

It even extends to the caregiver positioned between the patient and his family. The caregiver systematically isolates the patient from family members while swindling the patient's money and assets. Then, when the caregiver has depleted the estate, they have the patient's medications changed to more potent sedatives and then depose the patient into hospice services. **Please read more about this type of caregiver abuse at Kasemcares.org.

With six people surrounding Ms. Kab, we moved her through the door to where she was partially sitting up with her back leaning against the wall. Just the bottoms of her legs were still outside. Ms. Kab was quickly tired, which was too much for her.

As a titter-totter and a spinning top rolled into one, two people lifted Ms. Kab's legs, and the other four people pulled and turned Ms. Kab's body to where she was pivoting on her butt. As we turned her, her legs were pulled up higher to clear the door, and her body was once again allowed to lie flat.

Unfortunately, most respiratory-compromised patients cannot lie flat. It makes breathing more complex, and with Ms. Kab, because of her body mass, sitting up caused her belly to push up on her diagram, crushing her lungs.

We at least had Ms. Kab's entire body in the house. It was now just a matter of moving her to the bed, and fortunately, that part went smoothly. Until she snored,...

Families expect the peaceful passing of their loved one as if it were an equation with an exact final number that can not be changed. Rarely is that the case and Ms. Kab was no exception.

While the nurse and the family members bathed Ms. Kab, the doctor and I set up shop at the kitchen table. With our laptops open, we both tried to chart and finish our day as much as possible. Occasionally, a family member would appear and ask if we would like a drink or something to eat. Otherwise, the house was exceedingly quiet.

Dr. Chris ordered a little more comfort medication for Ms. Kab and then asked that I remove her from the BiPAP. By this time, Ms. Kab was non-responsive. She had gone to her happy place. The long day of leaving the nursing home/ALF, the transport home, the "slide her in" adventure, the bed bath, and the "comfort" medications left Ms. Kab drained.

I returned to the kitchen table to finish my charting, and within a few minutes, I was again joined by Dr. Chris, who proudly informed me that she had just pronounced Ms. Kab.

Seriously? That was quick. This was Dr. Chris's first home withdrawal. She was happy that at least what had started sketchy was finishing on the right note.

The quietness in the home was only disturbed by the click-click of the laptop keys, the swooshing of family members walking by, and the occasional flushing of the toilet,... until we heard a snore and a loud gasp, which seemed to have come from the direction of the patient. The dead patient

Dr. Chris and I looked at each other, frozen, with the "you go" and "no you go look" look. We both walked into the room to find Ms. Kab snoring, still quite alive, eight minutes after being pronounced dead.

## Holiday

Ms. Hobbs lived in a historic part of Florida in one of those not-so-idealistic trailer parks for those of low means, where several generations of family members live together. Her son and his wife lived with Ms. Hobbs, with her son picking up odd jobs and her daughter-in-law cooking and doing the household chores. I had visited Ms. Hobbs maybe half a dozen times. She was a funny, lively-spirited lady with the most adorable and protective little dog. I mention the dog because he would meet me at the back door each visit and tag along my side as I made my way to the front kitchen area where Ms. Hobbs would be sitting. As I approached the kitchen table, the little dog would turn and look at me as if to say, "That's far enough." When Ms. Hobbs would point to the dog treats on the table, I would grab a treat from the bag and hold it so the little dog would come closer. He took the treat as I spoke to him in a high-pitched sing-song way, and then he rolled over for a belly rub. It was pretty cute. That dog was her buddy and her everything.

Ms. Hobbs was always suspicious of hospice and for a good reason. At first, I thought she was talking about me and my visits, but she soon made it clear, when I inquired, that she was referring to the nurses inquiring about her code status. "They are always pushing me to sign that form." "What form, Ms. Hobbs?" "That yellow piece of paper that says I don't want anything done to me if I drop dead."

What Ms. Hobbs was referring to was a form that would be signed by her physician, in this case, the hospice physician, and signed by her stating that if her heart stopped or she stopped breathing, medical personnel would not intervene to help her. It is a "Do Not Resuscitate Order" (DNRO) stating that she would be allowed to die.

It is a patient's right to have a DNRO or not. And if you do have one, you can revoke it at any time, in writing, by physically destroying the form, by failing to present it, or by simply stating so at any time by the patient or the patient's health care surrogate.

Ms. Hobbs continued, "If something happens to me, I want everything done. I'm not leaving without a fight. "

Well, that will soon be tested.

From day one, all hospice patients are told that for any needs, concerns, or questions, they should call either their team or, after hours and on weekends, the hospice helpline. All their care will be provided and coordinated by hospice. These phone numbers are given to the patients as written on the front cover of their hospice binder and as magnets for their refrigerators. Some nurses go so far as to program the patient's phone for a speed dial number directly to hospice. Patients are often reminded that if they choose to go to the hospital without notifying hospice first, and it is not covered under their hospice services, they will be responsible for any bills generated from that hospital visit. How is a patient supposed to know what is and is not covered? So, that veiled threat works nicely.

And the way it is presented to the patient sounds like the perfect service. If they need something, they have someone to call 24 hours a day, seven days a week, just like a personal concierge service. However, what you may need or want is not always what you will get.

It was late one night when Ms. Hobbs was not feeling well. Her breathing was labored, and she felt as if she was coming down with a cold. She wanted to go to the emergency room at a local hospital. However, because of the warnings of incurring a bill, her family called the hospice after-hours number, as they had been directed to do so many times over, for advice. The hospice after-hours service advised them that Ms. Hobbs should come to the hospice center. The hospice center is a free-standing building with about 20 beds and round-the-clock nursing care. However, the family stated she wanted to go to the hospital for IV fluids and antibiotics. The after-hours nurse persisted and promised IV fluids and antibiotics would be available and given at the hospice center. Ms. Hobbs was transported to the hospice center.

Upon arrival, and shortly after that, the family asked when the IV fluids and antibiotics would be given. The nurse at the hospice center knew nothing about the promise made by the call center.

It is much like the admission process, where there is a case manager, a hospice referral nurse, and a hospice admission nurse, all feeding various pieces of information to a new patient. However, once you are admitted, you are now dealing with the team nurse, the after-hours nurse, and the hospice center nurse: different nurses with the same mode of operation. Tell the patient what they want to hear to get them to do as you wish.

The nurse at the hospice center told the family she would need to contact the doctor on call for the IV fluids. If the doctor gave the order for antibiotics, they would need to come from the pharmacy, which meant nothing would happen tonight. Meanwhile, she would provide Ms. Hobbs with some medication to help make her comfortable. By this time, it's about 1 am. Ms. Hobbs had been and was continuing to decline in how she felt and her alertness. Her family was anxious that she was not receiving the care she wanted and needed and was now insisting that 911 be called to take her to the hospital.

Of course, that request was met with pushback. After about another hour of the nurse trying to appease the family, the agreement was made for EMS to transport Ms. Hobbs to the hospital.

By this time, though, it was too much for Ms. Hobbs. She was already exhausted from a long day and the extra energy it took for her just to be able to breathe. Then, add in the stress of going to the hospice home and the "comfort" medications that were given to help her relax. She passed away just as the transport service arrived to take her to the hospital.

The DNRO would later be signed by the doctor, post-mortem, and included in the chart. Otherwise, upon reviewing this chart, the question would be, why was a patient who was a full code and in respiratory distress at the hospice home rather than at a hospital? Because it's cheaper for them to die at a hospice center than at a hospital, plus the bonus of the death being on hospice records, another win for hospice.

Fortunately, hospice only wins some of the time.

## The Final Road Trip Home

How many cemeteries do you pass as you go through your daily commute? Monuments to the dead, and we barely give them a second glance. Are they ignored consciously? Or is our DNA programmed with a survival instinct so strong that we cannot accept death or dying?

Your whole life has been summed up in this final moment. For some, it comes quickly; for others, it comes slowly. For some, it is as peaceful as a long-overdue nap that comes quietly in the night, or it is a painful struggle as if they were stuck underwater beneath a sheet of ice.

Ever since the time that we became mentally aware of our mortality, we know that death is only one heartbeat away. For most people, this thought is far from their everyday life. Briefly thought of, perhaps, when the birthday of an elderly loved one rolls around or when passing by an accident, thinking, "Hope they are alright, glad it wasn't me."

We all know death is a reality, but we do little more than prepare a will or living testament for that final moment. We plan births, weddings, careers, home buying, and retirement. Still, we neglect our final breath, our final heartbeat, our final goodbye. As if by ignoring it, it won't happen. It's only a myth in some faraway land. If only

Some patients do manage to pass away peacefully and in a place of their choosing, with loved ones at their side. One such patient was a gentleman I met with interstitial lung disease (ILD) - a most horrible disease that affects the lining of the lungs. It is a thickened wall of cells, a membrane encompassing the lungs.

I received a request from the home team to visit a newly admitted patient with ILD. Like so many people with this horrible disease, it can be misdiagnosed or not properly managed. These days, most primary care physicians try to treat all their patients themselves rather than send the patient to the appropriate specialist. Especially those managed care programs. "Managed Care." What appropriate wording because the physician is actually managing the financial aspect of care. A physician may only receive a set monthly amount to manage a patient. This type of care causes a conflict of interest. If the physician orders lab work, X-rays, or visits to other physicians,... these expenses impact the monthly amount the primary care physician receives to "manage" your care.

For older patients with ILD, it is frequently misdiagnosed as COPD until late in the disease's progression, when a simple breathing test (pulmonary function test) or a few history questions and a physical exam could have easily distinguished between the two physiologically drastically different diseases. While there is still no cure for ILD, symptom management is very different.

I felt relief as I pulled into the over 55 senior RV resort, which looked like so many other wintry residences hidden away like little gems. The hustle and bustle of the daily grind are left behind as I drive through the gates. Big, oversized cars and trucks are replaced with golf carts and three-wheel bikes, with a rear basket to carry home groceries from the store across the street. If you watched the movie "Cocoon," you know exactly what I'm talking about. And if you haven't, you should. It's a great movie, but dying is rarely that peaceful.

This day at the RV resort was similar to all the other days from mid-October until the end of April. This is the time of year when the snowbirds descend on their second home in the sun to escape the snowfields up north. Although, what was different was the couple I was about to meet.

They were here on their yearly trip to spend the winter in Florida, away from the snowy landscape of the North. When I first met Mr. L, he sat on the side of the bed, struggling to breathe. Each breath is measured and deliberate. Like so many I had seen before him, his whole existence focused on his breathing: this breath, the next breath, and the next—every minute of every day. And like so many others, he was being treated as if he had COPD, not ILD.

With ILD, the lining around the lung tissue becomes scarred, stiff, and thickened, and oxygen cannot readily move from the lungs into the bloodstream.

He had the usual oxygen ordered via a concentrator, which, as the name implies, supplies oxygen by "concentrating" the available oxygen in the room. An old, noisy, heat-generating electrical hog was tucked into the corner of his front room with his hospital bed. His nasal cannula was hanging from his face, and I could tell by the sound of the oxygen flow from his cannula that it wasn't much. His arms extended to support his weight, which we call the tripod position.

Someone in severe respiratory distress will try to support their upper body weight with their arms, whether sitting on the side of the bed or sitting up in bed. Their arms will be down at their sides, pushing on the bed, trying to extend the length of their torso, and pushing their shoulders up to expand the lung area. The muscles in their necks (accessory muscles) will be pronounced with each breath. All this extra effort to breathe uses more oxygen than the body has, which causes this catch twenty-two effect. The patient cannot get enough oxygen in the body. The body's natural reaction is to try and expand the lungs, which increases the work of breathing. All this extra effort uses more oxygen, so the body adjusts to try and increase oxygen flow into the lungs. And so the downward spiral begins.

The more oxygen you need, the more you struggle to get it. The more you struggle, the more your heart and respiratory rates increase, which uses more oxygen. You end up using more oxygen than you can obtain. The best thing to do in this situation is focus on breathing. Slow your breathing down, which in turn will decrease your heart rate. By changing your breathing, your heart will follow.

If you can decrease the work of these organs, the oxygen usage by the body will decrease. In the respiratory world, there is a saying, "Smell the roses, blow out the candles." -Pursed Lip Breathing If wearing a nasal cannula, breathing in through your nose (mouth closed) allows you to obtain as much oxygen as possible. Then, when exhaling through pursed lips, as if trying to blow out a candle slowly, slows the exhalation phase. Extending the inhale/exhale phase allows the oxygen/air mixture to stay in the lungs longer. This serves several purposes. It helps "push" the oxygen across the lung membrane into the bloodstream, "pops" open closed alveoli, helps splint the smaller airways, and allows slowing of the respiratory and heart rates by calming the body/mind. A simple technique that works

Mr. L could talk only one or two words at a time. I asked him if I could adjust his oxygen and start him on a nebulizer treatment. He gave me a look that said, "You have to ask?" With a smile and a wink to him, I immediately went to the oxygen concentrator to turn up the flow. His concentrator was already at a flow of 3 LPM on a 5 LPM max unit. This oxygen amount was nowhere near what his body was demanding. And the nebulizer he was given was a far cry from what he really needed.

After increasing his oxygen and starting him on a nebulizer treatment, I knew he needed to focus on slowing his breathing, which in turn would calm his body and heart rate. In a soft, calming voice, I asked him to close his eyes and focus on his breathing, with instructions for pursed-lip breathing and slow in and out. I asked his wife about his medication list as he continued his nebulizer treatment. Nothing was ordered for anxiety or to help with his work of breathing.

Mr. L was a DNR (Do Not Resuscitate), meaning he did not want any intervention in case his breathing or heart stopped. But he was still breathing, and his heart had not stopped, so I asked him if he wanted me to call 911. "What for?" His response was a statement, not a question. He knew that if 911 were called, they would place a breathing tube into his lungs, he would end up on a ventilator, and he would not make it back. He closed his eyes and dropped his head as if resigning to his fate.

I left him alone in thought as I reviewed his medications with his wife. At first, I could not quite keep up with her conversation as she went from talking about his medications to canceling a cruise. She was so overwhelmed. I remember thinking this would not go well if she could not keep it together. I asked if she had any family to help, and she mentioned her two daughters and sons-in-law in Maine, but no one was nearby to help.

After reviewing the medications that had been ordered for him, I called his hospice team, recommending that his oxygen be increased to 12 LPM via a high-flow nasal cannula and that he change to liquid oxygen as well as having it STAT ordered. Additionally, I recommended a little something for the anxiety as well as for the dyspnea.

I knew that changing the concentrator oxygen to liquid oxygen would immediately make a difference. I educated him on his disease process, how to conserve his energy with any activity, and how to best recover when he finds himself short of breath. Who was I kidding? He was short of breath all the time, so I knew he wasn't listening. He was exhausted. At that point, there was nothing else I could do for him but wait.

I called the liquid oxygen vendor and asked them to prioritize that order for Mr. L. It was delivered to his home in less than two hours.

The next day, I spoke with the wife, who reported that he felt much better since he started using the liquid oxygen. But that the other medications had not arrived yet. I asked if she or he had questions about our conversation during my visit. They had none. I said I would be out in a couple of days to re-assess him.

When I returned a few days later, I expected to see him more at ease, with less breathing effort. But he wasn't. His color was a little better, but he still seemed nervous. He was holding himself with his arms extended, sitting on the side of the bed. When I asked him how he felt, he said the liquid oxygen felt better in his lungs because it was cooler and smelled fresher. I asked about the oral medications and if they were helping or not.

The answer was, "I don't know; I haven't had any." My first thought was that the medications had not been delivered, but as I turned to speak with his wife, I saw the medications sitting on the counter unopened. The wife was afraid to give them to him, and he was afraid to take them because the label stated: "every four hours as needed."

Now, to some people who read "every four hours as needed" and think, "How hard can it be to figure that out? Take it when you need it." If only it were that simple.

Let's review: An elderly man is fighting for every breath he can get. This minute, this hour, all day long, every day. He was even afraid to move because it made his breathing harder. The wife was struggling with all the information, education, and the dying process of her husband. Neither knew what effect the medication would have on him nor did they know what "need" meant. And the warning label on the medication? Will the medication help or make him worse?

So, the medication sat unopened. I explained why each medication was ordered and reviewed the prescribing instructions and indications for use. It ultimately comes down to the patient whether to use it or not. However, I strongly suggested he use the medication as ordered, at least to try it once, or maybe even half a dose, whichever he felt comfortable doing.

As I finished up my visit, the team nurse arrived for her visit. I asked the nurse to review the use of the medications with the patient and his wife and answer any questions they may have regarding the medications' use. To say the same thing I had just said, hoping it would sink in.

I left, knowing this gentleman did not have many weeks left. I could only pray for a comfortable end.

A few days later, I revisited. Now, he looked much better. There was still the underlying struggle to breathe, but mentally, he was calmer. There was a change. The medications and change in oxygen helped a little, but reality had been accepted. However, his wife was still struggling to keep up with all of his needs. He was completely dependent on his wife for even the most basic activities of daily living (ADLs).

I continued to visit over the next couple of weeks. On one visit, I pulled up to Mr. L's home and was shocked to see him sitting just outside his front door with his wife. His wife had managed to thread the oxygen tubing outside so he could use it. I was almost in tears. He looked wonderful sitting in the fresh air and soaking up the Florida sunshine, although I told him the shocked look on my face was from the bright reflection of his neon pink T-shirt and green socks. During my next visit, he would get back at me as he commented on how he liked my "tan" on a morning I had used self-tanner on my face.

During a patient's upswing in clarity and energy, we call this a "rally." Each patient is different regarding when it happens, to what degree it happens, and the length of the rally. He was doing better because of the liquid oxygen and medication change. I also believe he looked forward to seeing his daughters and sons-in-law and taking the road trip.

I don't remember exactly when I learned of the road trip, but the plan was for the daughters and their spouses to fly to Florida, rent an RV, and drive Mr. L home to Maine. I remember standing in front of Mr. L, looking at him nearing the end of his life, being weak and tired. Too many thoughts flooded my mind. The logistics of such a trip were overwhelming to me, and I'm the organized one. My main concern was for Mr. L and his comfort. The liquid oxygen, the medication, the route to be taken, etc., the list was endless with all the "hows," "whats," and "what ifs."

I even envisioned them getting halfway home and Mr. L passing by en route. Did they stop to call the sheriff to report it or go to the nearest hospital? If they did, would Mr. L end up in a morgue three states away from home? Or if they continued on home, encountering a flat tire on the interstate and having AAA change the tire unaware of the circumstances in the RV. or the nor'easter about to hit (or approach) the East Coast.

I notified the hospice team and asked for assistance with an AAA Trip Ticket, someone to notify the hospice and send records to Maine, arrange for liquid oxygen for transport, check medications with a hard copy of the prescription, and other items. The hospice team had a manager in the office, a secretary, and a social worker to assist. The answer I received back from the home team was, "The family needs to do these things."

Now, which "family" would this be, the overwhelmed wife or the kids, 1500-odd miles away?

So, my next email was a little more specific. Would the social worker contact AAA and ask for a trip ticket? Would the team secretary make contact with the hospice in Maine? Has someone asked our DME company to arrange the liquid oxygen for transport? And please have the team physician write orders and H&P for the family to carry during travel if needed.

And the response to my email?

The social worker does not know how to get a AAA Trip Ticket.

The family needs to arrange for hospice.

The DME company said no.

And the physician, per the team, said, "Just take the pill bottles."

This back-and-forth lasted several days. During this time of going back and forth with the team about what needed to be done, the team nurse visited the patient's home to tell the patient and his wife that he was too fragile to travel and advised against it. She suggested the family come here to visit.

Yes, this man is fragile and at the end of his life stage. However, if he can sit on the side of his bed or lie in it, he can do the same in an RV. While I had my concerns about his travel, I certainly was not going to hinder his wish to go home, nor would I try to prevent it for the sake of being able to post that death on the hospice records. To them, it was/would be just another check in the box.

The hospice builds its need in the community on the number of admissions and deaths it can record. As sad as it is, it is true.

I was so angry about this whole situation, the lack of empathy from the entire team, and their lack of effort to help this man return home. It was to the point that I was embarrassed to even talk to the family about the travel plans because nothing was being done on this end. I was so ashamed of how this company touted care and compassion in public, but it was heartless and cruel behind the scenes. Is that harsh? True? Absolutely.

I circumvented the DME company by contacting the liquid oxygen supplier directly. We (RT and supplier) had a very good relationship, and they were willing to help even though they were a regional distributor and did not have any resources in the north. Additionally, they were willing to load a liquid canister in the RV and secure it for travel. I received two responses when I notified the hospice team that the liquid oxygen company was willing to help.

One: They would not pay the $250 deposit for the liquid oxygen canister.

Two: The social worker stated that oxygen could not be transported legally in an RV.

Are you kidding me? Seriously, I could not make this stuff up.

We are going to prevent a patient from going home over $250, and if the social worker who did not know how to get a AAA trip ticket (like calling AAA, visiting an office, looking it up online, etc.) knew the Department of Transportation's local, state, and federal regulations regarding the transportation of liquid oxygen across multiple state lines. If it were not so pathetic, it would be comical. This could be an SNL skit.

That one comment from the social worker was a complete roadblock for the hospice team. I spent nearly half a day tracking down the exact person in Washington who could tell me unequivocally, from a local, state, and federal perspective, the regulations regarding the transportation of liquid oxygen in a private vehicle through multiple states. We were nowhere close to the amount of liquid being transported that anyone would care about.

I finally emailed the entire team and told them that this gentleman would go home to Maine in an RV with his oxygen, whether we helped him or not, so please do what you can to help facilitate the move. Crickets. I gave the liquid oxygen company my personal debit card number to use as a deposit, which was never used. I wasn't about to tell the family about the deposit; they had enough to organize already.

During this time, the family was busy arranging with the hospice organization in Maine for continued care and delivery of needed equipment for the home, such as hospital beds, bedside tables, etc., as well as arranging flight plans for travel to Florida and the rental of the RV. Additionally, their daily life responsibilities would need to be arranged if they had children, time off from work, or pets. While we sat, twiddling our fingers, collecting Medicare money each and every day, Mr. L came one day closer to his final breath. I felt the urgency to get him home because I knew the window of opportunity was closing.

We were one week away from the family arriving from Maine and Mr. L's journey home to begin; at least that was the plan until I checked the weather. My heart sank as I saw the forecast for the end of the week.

There was a Nor'easter headed directly into the path of their route home. More than 1.8 million homes and businesses were without power, some areas expected more than a foot of snow, interstates and roads were closed due to coastal flooding, and some states declared an emergency.

I called the family and asked if they wanted to delay leaving. "No" was the answer. At that point, I was seriously concerned that something would happen en route if they left Florida. And the list of "something that would happen" ran the gamut from running out of gas or a flat tire to being trapped in a snowbank. Okay, maybe not a snowbank, but you get what I mean. Having never lived in an area that experienced such drastic weather, my imagination came up with various situations.

And what did not help my exaggerated thinking was the TV weather reports. They were so frequent and intense with the gloom and doom rhetoric that I became anxious just watching them. The storm was hundreds of miles away. Sometimes, I think the news channels make items more of an issue than they need to be just to keep viewers "hooked" for the next report.

How many times have you seen the live weather reports where the "journalist" has his body braced forward, leaning into the "blistering" 60 mph wind, only to end the segment before the cameras cut back to the studio. You see the "journalist" immediately stand upright, calmly walking away checking his phone? Or they pose themselves where the crosswinds create a wind tunnel, like between two buildings, only to take one step over to complete calmness. What happened to reporting the news and not creating it?

Also, I was letting go of one of my patients, who would now be out of my reach. Would the new hospice have someone to care for him as I would? Would they make sure he had his medications and oxygen as needed?

These were genuine concerns, as other patients have told me about how they are told to "ration" their oxygen use because they will only be given x amount of oxygen. Upon visiting one patient, before I could even finish introducing myself and the reason for my visit, he

He was desperately asking if I was going to make him cut back or ration his oxygen. Who would ever ask or tell a pulmonary fibrosis patient that they can only have so much oxygen or that they must ration their oxygen? That is absolute craziness and the added stress it places on a patient.

My final visit with Mr. L was on Monday. I gave my last traveling instructions to him and his wife and contacted the oxygen company to make sure all was well. The family would arrive the next evening, and the plan was to start Mr. L's trip home Wednesday morning.

Again, I checked the weather. The Nor'easter was slamming the eastern seaboard. I called the family and again asked about postponing. "No." I honestly don't blame them. I would move heaven and earth to get my mom home. I finally had to turn the cable weather channel off and just say a prayer.

I think they arrived home on Thursday night. The weather and traffic weren't as bad as they were portrayed on the TV news, or divine intervention escorted them home. I believe the latter.

Several weeks later, I would get a call from the family saying Mr. L had passed away peacefully at home surrounded by his family. I would hope for each of us this kind of final journey. I am very blessed to have met this couple, and it gives me hope that some families still put family first. You can have all the money and materialist things life has to offer. Still, it does come down to the final moments, the final loving touch, the final road trip home.

For every patient that makes it to their final destination on their terms, there are many, many more that do not.

Michelle Young Doers

## Three Days Dead

There are times in our lives when we find ourselves on a path that is not our choice—where the hard decisions are made at the crossroads of our lives. Do we take the safe, known route or the dangerous, unknown route? I'm not talking about "Do you want fries with that?" I'm talking about life-altering choices where we are mentally tested to make a choice that, once taken, we cannot undo.

At this intersection, as you take one step in either direction, the path behind you falls away, leaving you with only the path directly ahead. Now, on this path, you must see it through until the end, wherever that "end" takes you. As you make that journey, your integrity and beliefs will be tested along the way, as will your commitment to both.

And for some, the path has already been made; you don't know it yet.

For me, little did I know that that morning, my arrival at the hospice home would change the course of my life and career. A course that had already begun

Mr. Spykler was a 55-year-old man with recently diagnosed extensive small cell lung cancer. The lung cancer had spread throughout his entire body, attacking not only the delicate lung tissue but also his bones and spine. Every part of his body was in agonizing pain.

His breathing was not only affected by cancer, but the pain would have increased his heart rate, his blood pressure, and his breathing effort. He struggled in a balancing act, trying to decrease the pain with morphine, as prescribed by his physician, without further compromising his breathing. His underlying COPD from smoking only exacerbated the situation.

Living alone and in poverty, Mr. Spykler would drive himself to his doctor's appointment and the nearby pharmacy. There wasn't much anyone could do for him at this point. The constant pain and the struggle to breathe wore on his body. But he was not ready to give up the fight. He kept his appointments and organized his medications.

By organizing, I mean he would transfer the medications from the pill container supplied by the pharmacy to a daily pill minder (those plastic flip-lid containers holding a week's worth of daily medications in little individual compartments).

Everyone should know that any prescribed medications are to be kept in their original dispensing bottles provided by the pharmacy. The bottle contains all the information needed to identify the pills inside as well as the person for whom the medications were prescribed.

For the person at home, this method of using a pill minder is easy and helps a patient keep track of their medications. However, it should never leave the house, and we should inform patients of its proper use. If you must take your medications to an appointment, bring the whole bottle with all the identifying information labels attached. If you take just the pill minder and are in a car accident, would the paramedics know if the pills were yours, what type of medication, and in what dose? Or if you are pulled over for a faulty brake light or some other minor traffic violation by a deputy sheriff who notices the pill minder in the console while standing at your car window and believes the driver is acting "suspiciously"?

And that happened to Mr. Spykler on his way home from his doctor's appointment. I was not there during this incident, so I cannot speak of the details... only the outcome of his arrest.

I can only imagine the physical torment he felt from the disease within his body, the mental torment he knew of the air surrounding him, his struggle to breathe that air, and the cold, hard metal handcuffs digging into his wrists, clasping his arms behind his back.

With the adrenaline rushing through his body, his heart rate would have increased, thus using more oxygen. The more oxygen his body required, his respiratory rate would have increased. With the increase in his respiratory rate, anxiety would have set in, producing more adrenaline.

Increase in heart rate
Increase in oxygen demand
Increase in respiratory rate
Anxiety
Increase in Adrenaline

As you can see, this cycle can quickly spin out of control. And for Mr. Spykler, it must have felt like Hell, but Hell had not arrived yet.

The day after the arrest, Mr. Spykler was released and immediately taken to a local hospital emergency room. His last dose of morphine was the day before. His body would have been in excruciating pain, and his breathing labored. The withdrawal symptoms of morphine now compounded the pain and shortness of breath from lung cancer and COPD.

In the emergency room, they placed him on a bilevel-positive airway pressure (BiPAP) unit with a full-face mask. The full-face mask would cover his nose and mouth, forming a closed system between him and the BiPAP unit, similar to what fighter pilots would wear. The head strap buckled tight around the head to a mask with no holes, then attached to corrugated tubing.

To illustrate the mechanics of BiPAP within the lungs, consider a balloon. If you add air to a balloon until it is taut, that would be the inspiratory phase, or breathing in. Then, you deflate the balloon by half, the expiratory phase, or blowing out. Breathe in-expand, blow out-deflate. If you removed the BiPAP pressure, the balloon would nearly collapse, and the lungs would maintain only minimal pressure.

The BiPAP was now acting as his life support. With each breath, the BiPAP would supply, in this case, 100% oxygen compared to the 21% oxygen we breathe and an added inspiratory pressure of 16 cm H20. Then, upon exhalation, the pressure would drop to 10 cmH2O, allowing him to breathe out. With each breath he took, the BiPAP would help him breathe.

Additionally, I'm assuming at this point, the emergency room physician would have medicated him with some type of sedation, such as morphine, to ease the pain as well as his work of breathing.

Then comes the referral to hospice with a visit from a hospice admission nurse. The hospice admission nurse convinced Mr. Spykler of the comforts of hospice. I wasn't there, but I can certainly surmise that the usual "sale" spiel was along the lines of:

"we will make you comfortable"
"you'll have a private room"
"we'll help you get home"
"we will supply all your medications and medical equipment"

It's not only what the admission nurse says but the unanswered questions, the implied, the letting the patient and family fill in the blanks. After all, it's hospice—they help people. Here's the fallback for the admission nurses and the thought that must allow them to sleep at night and look themselves in the mirror: "It's what the patient/family wanted."

No, it's not

As I have stated elsewhere in this book, patients and families do not possess the knowledge to know all the pitfalls that await them around the corner. They are blindly led into a situation they have never encountered and can not imagine. They believe that hospice only does good and that a healthcare provider would not lie or mislead them. Nothing could be further from the truth. If you take nothing else from this book, please heed these words.

The hospice admission nurse who visited Mr. Spykler would tell me the next day of his condition. Noting that his BiPAP could be removed for 5–10 minutes to take his medications or have a sip of water, just after those few short minutes of being off the BiPAP, the EKG monitor (which was also monitoring his oxygen level and respiratory rate) would alarm due to his oxygen level being too low. He would then be placed back on the support of the BiPAP.

This nurse, knowing that Mr. Spykler could only come off the BiPAP for 5–10 minutes, had now arranged for transport from the hospital to the hospice home, which was thirty minutes away. The problem? When basic medical transport arrived at the bedside, the hospice nurse removed Mr. Spykler from the BiPAP or instructed the hospital personnel to remove the BiPAP and placed Mr. Spykler on a nasal cannula for oxygen at 6 LPM, which is about 44% oxygen.

The BiPAP that assisted his breathing, the 100% oxygen he received, and the splinting of his airways to allow air to move in and out of his lungs had all been taken away from him. No medication, no sedation.

Shortly afterward, en route to the hospice home, Mr. Spykler became extremely short of breath and panicky. The transport crew could do little more than place him on a regular oxygen mask at 100%. By the time he arrived at the hospice home, he was in total respiratory failure.

The nurses at the hospice home gave him 15 mg of morphine and 1 mg of Ativan to ease his suffering, but it was too late. His body was spent. And odds are, he most likely suffered a heart attack during the transport due to the lack of oxygen and extreme anxiety. When I saw him the next morning, he was mottled and had a respiratory rate of 3 breaths per minute. I was told the night nurse was in tears over the treatment of this patient. The cold, callous way this patient was managed, not only by the staff at the hospital but by the hospice physician who approved this plan and the hospice admission nurse who carried out the plan, was sickening.

The hospice admission nurse took it upon himself at the hospital to remove the BiPAP without a doctor's order. Although the hospice doctor may have approved the plan, he did not give an order to remove the BiPAP, which is considered "life-sustaining" by the FDA and requires a doctor's order. He indirectly murdered this patient.

All this was done with the intent of a speedy discharge from the hospital and admission into hospice. Also, how did the nurse obtain "consent to treat" from a medicated patient?

Does it matter that yesterday, Mr. Spykler was driving home from his doctor's office, and tomorrow, he'll be dead? Nope. Check in the quota box.

Mr. Spykler must have endured torturous suffering at the hands of those he entrusted with his life. Can you imagine the horror of being strapped tight to a stretcher and placed in an ambulance, hearing the doors slam shut, locking him in a metal tomb, cutting him off from the outside world, and, more importantly, from the machine he so desperately needed? Feeling as if he was being smothered and knowing that he was going to his death. Every second of that thirty-minute ride must have felt like an eternity in Hell.

I'm sure you ask, "Why would a patient agree to that treatment?" He didn't.

Who would sign up for that treatment? No one.

I completed an internal compliance report stating the facts surrounding the treatment of this patient. And how did the nurse discontinue life-sustaining support without a physician's order? A patient was killed for the sake of an admission.

Yes, this patient was killed for the sake of an admission, and that was the very last line of my compliance report: "Basically, we killed a patient for the sake of an admission."

I waited three days to write that report because my emotions were high. I was angry that someone could be that cold and callous to treat another person in such a manner. The admission nurse knew he could only survive 5–10 minutes off the BiPAP without having his oxygen level drop and having the feeling of being smothered. Still, the nurse took him off it anyway for that thirty-minute ride, also with no thought as to what the patient would need once at the hospice house. I could not sleep. I was physically ill for a week following this incident. 'What was the feedback I received from my manager about that report? One thing only: I should not have included the patient's name with that sentence because the compliance report would be included if any outside agency or entity requested that patient's chart. So, in other words, the message was that we can kill people; we just don't want others to know.

Little did I know at the time that this path I had chosen, or it chose me, was the beginning of my last eighteen months with hospice, and there would be more to come that I could not foresee.

## Death Through Chemistry

I awoke Thursday morning to hear the rain and distant thunder—such a soothing sound, tempting me to roll over and drift back to sleep. Early in the morning, this morning being 4 am is my favorite part of the day. It is dark, cool, and quiet. However, being off from work the day before, I knew I would need to start a little earlier this morning to clear out my emails and get ahead of the pre-weekend rush of discharges from the local hospitals.

Sorting through my email inbox, I found twelve emails flagged red, noting "high importance," with the same subject line: Vent Withdrawal. Over the last several years, that short two-word phrase has evoked an immediate sickening response in my body. I had come to dread those words.

As I read through the "high importance" emails, I realized the admission team had already planned a transfer of a patient from a long-term acute care center (LTAC) to one of the hospice houses for the removal of his life support this morning, which means in about an hour. There would be no way for us, a respiratory therapist, to facilitate the move or attend the withdrawal.

The Respiratory Therapist is responsible for evaluating a patient before the referral during the "education" process or at the referral from the hospital for the appropriateness of respiratory services within the scope of hospice.

After the respiratory assessment, a conference call would convene, and various medical professionals involved in the patient's care would discuss the patient's status and treatment plan.

Additionally, the R.T.s are responsible for a safe transfer from the facility, whether a hospital, an LTAC, or even from a patient's home to the hospice facility for discontinuing ventilatory support.

Now, we do not personally move the patient; we don't put them in the back seat of our car and deposit them on the doorstep of a hospice facility. We use an ALS (advanced life support) ambulance service.

We do have portable ventilators with built-in batteries. On the day of the transfer, we arrive at the patient's bedside to reassess the patient for any changes. Then, once admitted into service, we place the patient on our portable ventilator and give a report to the ALS transport team. The team then takes the patient to the hospice facility, where we meet with them again. We are then responsible for maintaining the ventilator for patient comfort, withdrawing the support, and supplying supplemental oxygen as needed.

How could we provide all that is required when no one notified us? We were also not included in the complex case conference call, which, by policy, is to be held before any withdrawal of life support. I emailed the main players of the conference call—the clinical manager, physician, medical director, and administrative director—stating we could not accommodate this procedure today due to no available staff and that we were not included in the conference call. I waited for the scathing replies.

Crickets.

Until my phone rang with a call from Dr. Scarecrow, the medical director. "What do you mean you can not do this withdrawal today?"

Without waiting for an answer, he continued, "How many R.T.s are working, and what are you doing? I want that patient at the hospice house at 1 pm. You can't tell me you're not doing this withdrawal."

At that point, I tuned him out. All I could envision was a six-year-old having a temper tantrum because he wasn't getting his way. He continued for another few minutes, alternating between making a statement and asking a question, although it was pieced together like a monologue. When he finally stopped to breathe, I calmly but firmly stated, "You need to calm down and do not talk to me that way. If you want to talk to anyone like that, it should be your admissions department, which is never organized to care for these types of patients properly. "

Let me be clear at this point. I respect every person and position within the healthcare system. Those who are generally behind the scenes, like the janitors and aides, have the most essential front-line jobs. They are the glue that keeps the rest of us on track and allows us to focus on our jobs. So when a physician wants to act and talk like he or she (and no offense meant, but I've only seen this behavior in men) is the end all and be all, that will get nowhere with me. Being a physician is a job description. Being a bank teller is a job description. Being an astronaut is a job description. I'm only guessing, but I would venture to say that nowhere in their job description does it say:
You can act like a jerk.
You can belittle others.
You may instruct others to work outside of policy.
You can give instructions to endanger others AND expect those instructions to be followed.
Human Resources would have a problem with those job duties, except at hospice.

He then asked, "Where are all the therapists?" I told him that there was only one therapist working today covering seven counties, which was Mindi, and she was doing a withdrawal two counties over.

So, this physician, who was determined to have his way, told me that he was going to call the medical director of the other affiliate where Mindi was performing an end-of-life withdrawal of life support to ask that she be released from that procedure to come and do his.

What??? I repeated his words back to him, "You are going to call another affiliate and ask them to send the therapist who is doing their organized end-of-life withdrawal of life support to come over and do yours?" He hung up.

A few minutes later, Mindi called, stating she had received a voicemail message from Dr. Scarecrow stating he had an emergency and needed her to call him as soon as possible. Since she was busy with a patient and their family, she called me requesting help with the call. I told her to ignore it and that I had already spoken to him.

The rest of that day was relatively uneventful. A conference call was scheduled for that evening to discuss the transfer of this patient for the next day and any outstanding documents needed, such as the capacity statement from a physician for this gentleman.

By the way, the attending physician at the hospital for this patient would not sign the terminality statement, which would indicate that this patient had a prognosis of six months or less, nor would he sign the capacity statements, which would indicate that this patient was not able to make decisions on his own.

During the conference call to finalize a treatment plan for this patient, it was mentioned that all the documents were completed. However, I knew that the attending physician refused to sign any of the documents, which left the question: who would be signing?

When I inquired who would sign the second set, a voice popped up and stated they were faxed to Dr. Scarecrow for his signature. What?? The hospice doctor

The hospice doctor, who had not seen the patient, was willing to do so. Let me say that again, the hospice physician, who had not seen nor visited this patient, was going to sign a capacity statement. He was willing to sign the capacity statement to proceed with the admission AND the withdrawal of life support.

So I asked, "How can he sign when he has not seen the patient?" After a brief silence, during which the silence alone can speak volumes, the clinical V.P. on the call spoke up and gave some convoluted, illogical explanation of the documents. She would later email me to explain further and state that she misunderstood the question. Right.

The next morning, I arrived at the hospital at about nine-ish and found my way to the patient's room. The room was empty except for the patient. The ALS transport was set for a 10 am pickup, or so I was led to believe. Where was the hospice admission nurse? Where was the bedside nurse who should have been packing this patient up for transport? *sigh*

I returned to the nurse's station to find the hospice nurse tucked in a corner, texting on her phone. "Brenda, Good morning. Are we ready to go into room 227? "I inquired.

She replied, being semi-startled, "Yes, I just need to admit him and hang these infusions." (Morphine and Verse)

"Okay, when can you do that?"

"Oh, anytime."

I wondered if my thought of "Well then, what the heck are you doing sitting there?" showed on my face.

I turned and went back to the room. Just outside the room in the hallway, I unpacked my portable transport ventilator and waited for Tina to arrive. Tina was a new-hire therapist; I was to shadow her as she performed her first ventilator withdrawal.

We could not place the patient on the hospice ventilator until he was admitted since he was not our patient, and I had no legal or professional right to treat him. So I checked and responded to various other emails, including one to the care team at the hospice house, stating that the patient was a little restless but otherwise stable.

Finally, Brenda made her way down the hall, juggling the two infusion pumps, electrical cords, medication tubing, and medication bags in her arms. She walked straight into the room, squeezing her robust frame between the foot of the bed and the wall. Then, with a side shimmy, she scooted between the A/C grill along the wall and the bed railing, making it to the far side of the bed, enabling her to deposit the items on a table.

She then reversed her movements to return to the door to don her gown and gloves. The patient was on contact isolation for C-Diff, which required anyone entering the room to wear a protective gown and gloves. Brenda had already dusted the bed frame, rails, walls, and A.C. vent with her street clothes, so it was a moot point.

After a few minutes, Brenda reappeared in the doorway. As she removed her protective gown and gloves, I asked her to check on the ALS transfer ETA since they should have arrived by now. "I have them on will-call," she replied.

"Will-call? It's 10:30, and they should have been here now. We do not set up a transfer of a ventilator patient on will-call; we could be bumped all day." My frustration was beginning to show. By now, we were about 20 minutes past the time the transfer should have started.

She started the infusions (morphine and versed), and she headed back to her computer to admit this patient.

As I watched her retreat down the hall, I could only close my eyes and shake my head. Nothing changes. You would think a nurse would know that the patient should be admitted into hospice services before starting any medications on a patient. She had Morphine and Versed being administered to a patient who wasn't even our patient. And if that was not enough, no one from the hospital staff stopped her. She could have gone into ANY room and hung those medications without anyone noticing. What would be the difference? This patient, that patient, the patient three rooms down...at this point, it made no difference; none of those patients or this patient was a hospice patient at this moment.

Think about that for a moment; a lady in street clothes can walk into a patient's room, administer two different medications for sedation, leave them running into the patient through an I.V., and walk out of the room, and no one says a word or notices.

At about that time, the bedside (hospital) nurse appeared. He was headed into the patient's room. I asked him when was the last time the patient had had a trial wean from the ventilator.

"Que?"

I asked again and received the same answer.

Okay, my fault. I should have asked the bedside respiratory therapist this question or asked the question in Spanish.

So I asked: "Has the patient received any sedation this morning?" I only received a puzzled look.

"Sedation, how much?"

"Ah, two hours."

"Yes, but how much?"

"Right now."

" No, No, No," I said as I saw him holding a clipboard-like tray with a syringe precariously perched upon it.

"Sedation?" I said to him, motioning to the syringe.

"Of course."

An unlabeled syringe filled with a clear fluid is placed back into the syringe wrapper. As I looked at him, I raised my eyebrows, and without moving my head, I allowed my eyes to look again at the syringe and back at him.

He then questioned me, "Que?"

I just motioned "no" to him and waved him off.

The patient did not need any more sedation, with two IV infusions of sedation already being administered. How can this nurse work in a hospital with mainly, if not all, English-speaking patients and not be able to communicate with them? I can only surmise that the patients assigned to him would be those who could not communicate. Although that little plan would only work if there were no patient emergencies or, maybe, like a fire, communication between staff and patient was a matter of life and death. Or something insignificant... like medications. Right.

Brenda calls me from the nurses' station, echoing down the hall, "He's admitted now."

Finally.

The hospital respiratory therapist in the adjoining room came over when he saw me at the doorway.

"Can I give you a hand?" He asked. I looked over at Tina; she was to be the lead on this morning's withdrawal. However, she was now so nervous about the whole situation and what she had just witnessed that she was just about in tears. I should have been shadowing her, but now she has declined to participate. I could not blame her. "Yes, please," I answered as the three of us entered the room to place the patient on our transport ventilator.

We exited the room to see transport unpacking their gear. Thank goodness this show can be on the road.

The EMS guys exchanged glances, then looked back at me, and one said, "He is on a vent?"

"Yes," I replied, "it is our transport vent, but if you're uncomfortable using it, you can use yours."

"We are BLS, not ACLS, and we cannot take ventilator patients."

Brenda, who had followed them down the hall, quickly chirped in, "I told them ACLS, you said ACLS, that's what you told me to order. I ordered ACLS". Classic. I'm sure she did.

It's one of those moments when you wonder, "What else could go wrong?" Tina and I returned to our little spot across from the patient's doorway on the other side of the hallway. I mentally retreat to my happy place while still focused on any sounds or alarms coming from my ventilator. Nothing. At least the patient was calm and quiet.

What should have started at 10 am was now almost 1 o'clock.

Finally, the ACLS unit arrived, and we were on our way, or at least I thought so.

Brenda and the bedside nurse walked swiftly back from the nursing station to the room. The bedside nurse was again carrying his clipboard as a tray with a filled syringe on it. As I looked between Brenda and the syringe, Brenda said, "I asked him to give the patient a little something for the road."

I said, "You have two infusions going; use them."

"Oh, I always have the nurse give them a little something, and I have increased his versed," Brenda said as both nurses turned and entered the room.

The patient is no longer the hospital's patient, so the bedside nurse should not give ANY medications.

My thoughts were interrupted by the paramedic asking me what infusions were running. I told him morphine and versed.

He then asked, "And what is that other nurse giving?"

"Ativan"

His eyes widened, and he asked, "Why?"

"Exactly"

Nothing changes. How much I complain about the lack of education the hospice nurses receive regarding medications does not matter. And it is their show at this time. If the patient is stable respiratory-wise, I can only say so much. In their judgment, the patient needed ativan in addition to the morphine and versed already in place.

We arrived at the hospice house without incident. It was time. The physician spent time with the patient and family and allowed the family to have time alone with the patient. There was just one outstanding question: where was the other capacity statement?

Well, it turned out that the physician at the hospice house was told to (as in "you will") sign the capacity statement by his boss, the hospice medical director.

So apparently, once it was mentioned on the conference call, for all to hear, that the medical director intended to sign the capacity statement even though he had not assessed the patient, the buck was then passed to the medical director's underling.

How many other patients' capacity statements were signed by a hospice physician who had not personally assessed the patient? These capacity statements are signed on the report given by a nurse fulfilling her quota.

The hospice house physician did as he was told to do. He signed the capacity statement after he assessed the patient's drug-induced cocktail of morphine, versed, and ativan cognitive status.

In private, I questioned the physician about the capacity statement. I asked if he found it odd that the primary care physician did not sign either of the documents. And still, he remains on record as the patient's primary care physician.

He stated that that physician, like others, remains on the record "even though they never see their patients again." I asked why the organization allows this, and the answer was, "Because they are a good referral source."

I said, "That's illegal."

"Yes, it happens all the time," came his response.

"It happens all the time." It was a recurring theme.

He continued to express his concerns, but after he had reviewed the patient's medical records and since there was a capacity statement in the chart already signed by the patient's hospital physician, he felt "relatively okay" with signing the capacity statement.

Relatively okay?

It is relatively okay to sign a capacity statement to decide to euthanize this patient.

I asked, "How do you know that the other physician doesn't have their reason for signing the capacity or DNRO when the patient's primary care physician would not sign either?"

"I don't." was the answer from the hospice physician.

At this point, I had two choices. Refuse to participate in the withdrawal of life support from this patient or assess my gut feelings and moral/ethical compass.

If I refused to withdraw the life support, that would mean the hospice doctor would be forced to remove the breathing tube from the patient. The breathing tube, known as an endotracheal tube (E.T.), extends from just outside the mouth, through the back of the throat, and down into the lungs. These tubes have a balloon on the distal end that must be deflated before removal. In addition, other safeguards must be followed to avoid injury to the patient or needless suffering. The hospice physician would not know this procedure since this is not his area of expertise, and on one occasion of an extubation, he announced: "Just cut the pilot balloon." That one statement speaks volumes about the lack of knowledge. Anyone who practices this method does not know basic 101 ET care or patient safety.

I felt I had no choice. I was put in the position of having to decide whether to let the patient potentially suffer at the hands of an inexperienced physician or do the procedure myself. I was angry about being put in this situation. I was angry at the physician for not taking a stand. And I was also angry at myself for not stopping the transfer back to the hospital.

I told the hospice physician, "This is all on you. You own this situation. It's on you, and I will not back you up. "

With the patient's mom and other family members at the bedside, along with the physician and care team, I disconnected the patient from life support.

Kevin never took another breath.

*Side note - Dr. Scarecrow mentioned earlier in this patient's story, was fired month's later for allegedly arriving one morning at the hospice office - Drunk.

## Court of Public Opinion

Tuesday August 14th, 2018

Following the removal of life support from Kevin, I wrote an email to my manager and our medical director stating that I would no longer participate in end-of-life withdrawal of life support. I cited my reasons as the blatant disregard for patient safety, illegal activities, inexperienced nursing care, and overuse of sedation.

Wednesday August 15th, 2018

We received a referral for Ms. Sage, who would arrive from "out of county," meaning this patient was not currently in this hospice's service area. Individual hospice organizations provide hospice services, and the state licenses each hospice to operate within certain geographical regions, such as by county.

So, suppose a patient wishes to use the services of a hospice but lives outside the hospice's service area. In that case, the receiving hospice only knows the patient through the paperwork provided by the sending facility or verbal communication from the sending facility. No one from the receiving hospice would have seen or assessed the patient. The information that would have been reported on the patient would have come from the out-of-county hospital case manager and the bedside nurse, all with their agenda.

Patients from out of the country typically present with numerous problems although they are stable and transferred for reasons such as being closer to family. However, when a patient is transferred from out of the county into service for end-of-life discontinuation of life support, the issues and concerns multiply tenfold.

The hospice physician asked the admission department to assure her that the patient would arrive with a double-lumen PICC. We would need two IV lines for the sedation since two medications would be used: morphine and Ativan. The patient arrived with one IV line, and that IV had an infusion of propofol going into this patient.

As the physician instructed the nurse to discontinue the propofol, I recall that propofol wasn't mentioned by the admitting nurse, only that the patient was unconscious and non-responsive.

And yes, that would be correct, given the propofol use. But why was propofol used if this patient had been unconscious for the last several months? Was she unconscious due to medication or truly unconscious from brain injury? Again, I said nothing.

Thursday, August 16th, 2018

I received an email from the Chief Compliance Officer, who also happened to be the Chief Clinical Officer (how convenient it is for an organization to have both of these critical positions rolled into one wolf watching the chickens), asking for an explanation of the allegations I made in the August 14th email to my manager, which I knew was really a fishing expedition. They were aware of everything I said; they just wanted to know how much I knew.


Monday, August 20th, 2018

In a two-page memo to the corporate clinical officer, I cited the EthicsPoint entry I completed on the previously mentioned Mr. Spykler. My last line of that report was, "Basically, killing a patient for the sake of an admission." I went on to state that I have little faith that any of this will matter other than to satisfy the curiosity of the legal department about to what extent an employee knows and will say.

I continued to state how the admission nurses misrepresent the patient's condition to gain an admission and bend to the care partner's needs (the hospital or LTAC wants the bed for a higher reimbursed patient) over the patient's best interest or safety. I went on to cite over fifteen items ranging from patients being discharged home without equipment and/or medication in the home, admission nurses being pressured by the organization by a quota system that jeopardizes patient care and safety, staff physicians signing capacity statements on patients they have not assessed, patients/families not being given a choice to choose their attending physician, nurses withdrawing life-sustaining ventilator support without a physician's order to gain an admission, nurses signing physician/ANRP signatures on orders when the physician/ARNP is on vacation, and In my opinion, admission nurses planned with the family even though the patient has the capacity and does not want hospice and to include inexperienced nurses who are doing life support admissions with medication infusions which, in my opinion, euthanized a patient with improper use of sedation.

Monday August 27th, 2018

I was summoned to a meeting with my manager and the Chief Clinical Officer (CCO) to discuss my complaints. However, the Associate Vice President of Human Resources opened the door when I arrived at the meeting room.

After a few minutes of small talk, another lady who was an aide to the chief clinical/compliance officer entered, shortly followed by the chief compliance officer.

To my best recollection, the CCO started by responding to a statement I made in my email regarding "satisfying the curiosity of the legal department." She wanted to assure me that this meeting was to clarify my concerns so they may be completely investigated and corrective action taken if needed. "If needed."

I stated that I had little faith that anything would come of this meeting since nothing was done in light of Mr. Spykler. "I didn't know anything about Mr. Spykler." The CCO stated.

She had been with the company for three years, but this incident happened last year. "You're the Chief Compliance Officer who oversees all EthicsPoint entries. How do you not know about this one?" "My staff did not give it to me." An EthicsPoint entry that accuses a company of killing a patient and is not given to the CCO for review? "No," so she claimed no knowledge of such a report and was willing to throw her staff under the bus. And if we gave her the benefit of the doubt that she did not know about it at the time, she knows now, as of 13 days ago. Would that not be the first discussion.? An employee accuses a company of killing a patient, and there is no further discussion. And the employee who accused the organization of killing a patient is sitting right in front of you. Nope. It was dropped.

The item that gained the most attention from her was the admission nurses' quota expectation statement. She tried to convince me there were no quotas, only expected productivity. According to her definition, admission nurses were expected to visit 5-6 patients daily to educate them on hospice services. I said, "No, that's not how it is. The nurses are expected to visit 10–12 patients daily for educational purposes and meet a 2-admissions-per-day quota. If they work 12 hours, their quota is 3. We must have had a ten-minute back-and-forth on this one subject. I knew what was what, and she would not convince me to get into the corporate line.

And if that was not enough, she proudly stated that a patient's average length of stay is less than seven days. That must be a comforting thought for our patients since most of our patients are admitted into service with a prognosis of six months or less. I'm unsure if the emphasis should be on six months or the "less" part. I guess it all depends on which side of the medicine cup you stand, sit, or lie.

The other bane of contention was the reality of the care our patients received. At one point, she said she knew exactly how our patients were treated because she was in meetings all day, every day, talking about such care. Meetings. At what point do you know the reality of bedside care while sitting in a boardroom? I stated that the corporate impression of care and the bedside reality of care are two different things. She said, "I can read a chart and know exactly what happened." No, by reading the chart, you only know what someone wants you to think happened, not what really happened. It was as if she was trying to brainwash me, that if she said it enough times, it would make it true. But naive me, she knew exactly what was happening, and she was pushing that agenda.

Now, at this moment, for all those times I stood and watched but said little, for the situations in which I participated but did not fully approve, for all the times I pushed back against the system for what was happening and nothing changed, it was as if the last seven years of being silent had finally bubbled to the top. I looked her straight in the eyes and flatly stated, "You must be delusional."

You would think that if an employee tells the number two person of a multimillion-dollar organization in an opposing conversation that "you must be delusional," that would be grounds for dismissal right then and there. Nope. Because if they did, the whole Pandora's box of allegations I made about patient safety and illegal activities would now be on public display in what they feared would be a potential lawsuit.

Tuesday, September 7th, 2018

No, they waited another week. And what was the supposed reason for my termination? I worked on my day off, August 15th. Yes, it was my day off, and I worked to help a newly hired employee and a patient. If it was such an offense, why didn't my manager state that when I called her on the 16th to add three hours of clock time to my payroll sheet, and she thanked me for helping? An employee was terminated for working on her day off 24 days ago or complaining about patient care, unsafe practices, and illegal activities 11 days ago.

You be the judge.

## Letter to Department of Health Services - Washington

13 Dec 2018
Ms. Seema Verma  Administrator - Center for Medicare and Medicaid Services
Room 445-G Herbert H. Humphrey Building
200 Independent Avenue SW, Washington, DC 20201

Re: Competitive Bidding Product Categories - Ventilators

Working in the healthcare field as a Respiratory Therapist for over thirty years, I thought I had seen it all until I worked outside the walls of the hospital and within the walls of a patient's home.

During my recent seven year tenure with hospice, I had a bird's eye view to the reckless nature that has evolved in the home care environment.  I will summarize some practices that I witness first hand by hospice and other homecare agencies specific to 'Life Sustaining' equipment implemented within the home settings. Life Sustaining, meaning without the needed equipment (ventilator or continuous-use BiPAP) life would not be sustained. This classification of 'Life Sustaining' is designated by the FDA and Medicare.

Please think about that for a moment - without this equipment life would not be sustained.

Now think about the patient in their home using a run of the mill BiPAP unit intended for sleep apnea and for use at night only. These type of units do not contain an alarm or a back-up battery, however they are used as 'life Sustaining' equipment.

Imagine your child with muscular dystrophy confined to a bed and dependent on life sustaining equipment for his every breath. The equipment provided has no alarm to notify you if he becomes disconnected nor does it have a battery back up in case of down power, as what happens with Florida thunderstorms. As a parent, you depend on the equipment provided to do the job it is intended to do. However, when improper equipment is placed in the home, that faith is missed placed as was the case with Cheryl - a parent of a child with MD. She would lay awake at night, just to hear him breath. This breath, then the next not knowing if and when the 'Life Sustaining' equipment would fail.

Or the husband whose wife was had ALS and was dependent on life sustaining equipment. Again without the back-up battery, during the night when electrical power was lost, the only thing that saved her life was the alarm on the oxygen concentrator. Which in itself is ironic since she was being mismanaged and did not require oxygen, but it was the oxygen concentrator that saved her.

I give you these examples to illustrate what happens when the lowest bidder is used and improper (cheap) equipment is placed in the home without proper oversight. As a Respiratory Therapist, I can recognize the dangers and safe guard these types of patients while choosing the appropriate equipment. These patients really do not have a voice, we (you and I) must be their voice to say - Proper care trumps profits.

These, and many more examples, are happening everyday across our Nation within the homes of our neighbors, friends and families.

While the healthcare industry may have it's standards, certifications and regulations, it is sorely lacking in direct oversight when it comes to homecare services. Without competent professionals, patient care and safety are compromised in an effort to maximize profits.

We could equate this to 'Life Sustaining' equipment within the hospital setting. Where in the hospital are you going to find patients on this type of equipment? Only in the Intensive Care Unit (ICU) where the nursing and therapist acuity level and education is elevated to a higher degree within a controlled environment with all the alarms and monitors. Then why would we put these same types of patients at home (uncontrolled environment) without the proper equipment nor the Respiratory Therapist to maintain these patients? It's crazy.

Hospital - All the bells and whistles.
Home - Fend for yourself.

Same patient, same disease, same needs - different standards.

In closing, let me borrow a partial quote from Astronaut John Glenn
"... if you were getting ready to launch and knew you were sitting on top of 2 million parts, all built by the lowest bidder on a government contract.'

So, when someone says 'it's not rocket science" - yes, yes it is.

Respectfully submitted,
Michelle Doers, B.S., R.R.T., C.P.F.T

## For Love or Money - Money

America Today

America saw its first hospice in 1974 - Connecticut Hospice - founded in Branford Connecticut.

By 1979, The U.S. Health Care Financing Administration (HCFA) assesses 26 hospices nationwide for cost-effectiveness, as well as what hospice is and what it should provide.

In 1983, President Reagan signs the Medicare Hospice Benefit into law.

Then in 1993, under President Clinton's health care reform proposal, hospice is a nationally guaranteed benefit accepted as part of the U.S. health care system.

Today, hospice is big business backed by Medicare dollars with each hospice fighting to control their service area. Before a hospice organization can open its doors, some states require a Certificate Of Need (CON) - incidentally, the initialism forms an appropriate acronym - in which it wants to operate.

For those hospices already operating in a given area, they will petition the state to deny a request from such an interloper to maintain their monopoly.

As an example, public records show in 2015 a 218-page petition was filed to the State of Florida's Agency for Health Care Administration by LifePath Hospice of Hillsborough county to deny a CON to two applicants citing "both applicants are sponsored by hospitals that serve as a primary source of referrals to LifePath". Those applicants being West Florida and Suncoast BayCare. This request was upheld.

However, in May 2016 Seasons Hospice & Palliative Care of Tampa was approved to open a hospice service within Hillsborough County.

Then in late September 2018, LifePath announced the opening of a 16 bed unit within Tampa General Hospital, the third-largest hospital (1011 licensed beds) in Florida. The top two being Jackson Memorial in Miami with 1493 beds and Florida Hospital Orlando with 1398 beds. Rounding out the top five are UF Health Shands Hospital in Gainesville with 895 beds and Orlando Regional Medical Center with 888 beds.

LifePath managed to position itself, by aligning with Tampa General Hospital, in a way that mirrored their opposition to other hospices as outlined in the court petition.

This is the same hospice that defended itself against a lawsuit brought forth by a former social worker, who worked for LifePath for over twenty years.

You can read more

https://caselaw.findlaw.com/us-11th-circuit/1886962.html

https://www.washingtonpost.com/business/economy/terminal-neglect-how-some-hospices-fail-the-dying/2014/05/03/7d3ac8ce-b8ef-11e3-96ae-f2c36d2b1245_story.html?utm_term=.27a0f2054772

https://www.wtsp.com/article/news/investigations/chapters-hospice-denies-state-investigation/292187663

Excerpts From News Report

"According to the lawsuit, in 2008, LifePath and Good Shepherd Hospice were audited and found to have 20 to 40 percent of patients who were not appropriate for the care. As a result, 600 patients were dropped from these local hospice centers because they no longer qualified. Also as a result of the 2008 audit, the organization had to repay Medicare more than $2 million."

https://www.wtsp.com/article/news/investigations/does-hospice-push-people-into-program-to-make-money/67-308161789

"Michael Murphy is a prime example. Murphy's mother got sick and needed some hospital care. But then, he says a hospice nurse approached his mother several times and convinced his family to move her into the Melech Hospice house.

"I am unaware to this day how she could have qualified to go to hospice," Murphy told us. After just three weeks, hospice also determined she no longer qualified. The bill to Medicare for three weeks was $40,000.

"It's like a salesman. Try to sell them on the hospice's house," says a former hospice nurse "They always wanted to keep the hospice house full -- no empty beds."

## Well, If They can do it,......

No matter the name, the potential for wrong doing is there.

- Compassionate Care Hospice Group agreed to pay $2.4 million to resolve allegations that its subsidiary, Compassionate Care of Atlanta, paid kickbacks to five physicians to get them to refer patients and certify them as eligible for hospice services. The company then billed Medicare and Medicaid for those patients, the lawsuit alleged. (Justice.gov)

- Guardian Hospice, which provides services in the Atlanta area, agreed to pay $3 million to resolve allegations it billed taxpayers for patients who were not terminally ill. (Justice.gov)

- Hospice Compassus, with facilities in the Atlanta area, agreed to pay $3.9 million to settle claims that it billed the federal government for patients who were not terminally ill. (Justice.gov)

- Serenity Hospice of Dublin, whose locations include Peachtree City, agreed to pay more than a half-million dollars after it was accused of submitting claims for ineligible patients. (Justice.gov)

- Hospice of Arizona along with American Hospice Management, which had locations in Atlanta, Cumming, Snellville and McDonough, agreed to pay $12 million to resolve allegations that its Arizona unit made false claims to Medicare for ineligible services. (justice.gov)

- Altus Healthcare & Hospice of Atlanta known as AAH Hospice, agreed to pay $555,572 to resolve allegations it submitted false or fraudulent claims to Medicare. (FBI.gov)

- Southerncare, which has 99 locations in 15 states, agreed to pay $24.7 million after the government accused it of charging Medicare for patients who didn't qualify. (Justice.gov)

- Chemed Corp and Vitas Hospice Services agree to pay $75 million to resolve False Claims Act Allegations relating to billing for ineligible patients and inflated levels of care. (Justice.gov)

Potentially the largest hospice case, alleging as much as $200 million in false claims, is pending before the 11th Circuit Court of Appeals here. That case involves AseraCare, which operates hospices in several states, including Georgia.

The AJC is interested in hearing from those who have had family members in hospice care in Georgia. Email  doctors@ajc.com

As of June 2019 there are over 600 published reports of criminal wrong doing on the Department of Justice website concerning hospice organizations.

Say what??  Can we break down that last sentence?
      - 600 published reports
      - Criminal wrong doing
      - Department of Justice
      - Hospice

AND That's The Ones We Know About!

Any day of the week you can do a google search of hospice lawsuits and the search results know no geographical boundaries.

- A Gainesville-based hospice program with some operations in Jacksonville, Orange Park and Palatka has agreed to pay roughly $5.1 million to resolve complaints it knowingly billed the government for unnecessary services, submitting false claims to Medicare and Medicaid for medically unnecessary care. (justice.gov)

- Texas - Brad Harris, who founded Novus Health Care Services in Frisco, Texas, wanted to speed up as many deaths as possible in order to maximize profits was indicted in a $60 million Medicare fraud scheme. Communications between Harris and nurses included texts like "You need to make this patient go bye-bye." An FBI affidavit alleges that he made comments like "if this f— would just die" and said in one meeting that he wanted to "find patients who would die within 24 hours." (justice.gov)

- South Carolina, Jim Carlen, who was suffering from Alzheimers but could walk with a walker and speak, died days after entering a hospice as an in-patient because his diabetes and blood pressure medicine were withdrawn and replaced with lethal doses of morphine and klonopin. (washingtonspost.com)

- In Maryland, Beverly Gargiulo, 62, of Pylesville, was admitted to the hospital for ulcers, was mistakenly advised to get hospice care, and then was given excessive doses of pain-killers and died according to a family lawsuit. A jury awarded the Gargiulo family more than $900,000. (washingtonpost.com)

- California a 31 yr old woman whose boyfriend tried for 10 hours to reach hospice as she gurgled and turned blue. (time.com)

- New York family called repeatedly for middle-of-the-night assistance. They did not receive care as the hospice workers were unaware of who was on duty. (time.com)

- In Michigan, a dementia patient moaned and thrashed at home in a broken hospital bed, enduring long waits for pain relief in the last 11 days of life, and prompting the patient's caregiver to call nurses and ask, "What am I gonna do? No one is coming to help me. I was promised help at the end." (time.com)

This list is only a few of hundreds, if not thousands, of complaints and lawsuits filed every year against hospice. These are not rogue hospices, this has become common place for too many hospices.

They say they have 24/7 care available, however they fail to say that care on the weekend, Holiday or after hours will be mostly, if not all, only be phone. The help will not come. But they will certainly bill Medicare in fraudulent claims.

The over promise and under delivery is the mantra of hospice. The services offered by hospices throughout the country vary by State and then further vary by the individual hospice organization's own service and admission policy, however there are basic services they must provide by Medicare standards.

## Office of The Inspector General Report

In a report released by the Office of the Inspector General in July 2018, cites: "hospices do not always provide needed services to beneficiaries and sometimes provide poor quality care. In some cases, hospices were not able to manage effectively symptoms or medications, leaving beneficiaries in unnecessary pain for many days".

The OIG report continued:

"OIG also found that beneficiaries and their families and caregivers do not receive crucial information to make informed decisions about their care. Further, hospices' inappropriate billing costs Medicare hundreds of millions of dollars. This includes billing for an expensive level of care when the beneficiary does not need it. Also, a number of fraud schemes in hospice care negatively affect beneficiaries and the program. Some fraud schemes involve enrolling beneficiaries who are not eligible for hospice care, while other schemes involve billing for services never provided."

"Lastly, the current payment system creates incentives for hospices to minimize their services and seek beneficiaries who have uncomplicated needs. Within each level of care, a hospice is paid for every day a beneficiary is in its care, regardless of the quantity or quality of services provided on that day."

***PLEASE read that last paragraph again.

It is 2020,...has anything changed with the payment system to hospices?   No.

## Take Away

Hospice does not need more regulation; it needs more direct oversight. We can no longer allow the fox to watch the hen house. A hospital, home care, or hospice is not doing the patient a "favor." The patient is doing them a favor by employing them as a service provider.

In closing, despite its shortcomings and propensity for ill gains, there is a need for this type of service when done right.

Until we as a society recognize that a person's right to die is basic and fundamental, these issues of dependency on a broken system will continue. The use of a hospice-type service cannot be made out of a patient's financial status nor the financial gain of family members, hospitals, or the hospice.

We owe it to our fellow men, our community, and the next generation to be our brother's keeper. With such well-documented fraud and abuse of the system at the hands of the hospice, we must also ask why something has not been done. Do the lawmakers not know, or do they know and still do not want to take action?

We have managed to turn what started as warm, affectionate love into cold, hard cash. Any attorney would warn you not to make any life-altering decisions based on emotions, such as buying or selling a home or making other significant decisions in the wake of the death of a loved one. But when it comes to your end-of-life decision, we are given the grim prognosis of facing death and then expected to make a literal life-or-death decision within hours.

Choose wisely.

## Further Explanation

*Ms. Minnie*
(From page 25)

Six Minute Pulse Oximetry

Pulse oximetry is a small device placed on the end of a finger to gauge a patient's oxygen level. In the home setting, it is a battery-operated device roughly one inch across by two inches long. It opens like a clamshell and closes over the finger. Within the space where the finger sits, a thin beam of light is emitted from inside and through the fingernail. On the underside of the finger pad is a receptor that receives light. The receptor then calculates a rough estimate of the oxygen levels based on the color of the light it receives after passing through the finger. Many patients have these items in their homes since they are readily available over the counter at most local pharmacies or online. I'm not a fan of patients having this item in their home for use, nor of the nurse who also uses this device for several reasons.

First, it is a rough ballpark estimate, not an exact measurement of the oxygen level within the blood. It is one piece of the overall picture of the patient's condition. Its accuracy is affected by blood circulation when the hand is cold, improper placement, ability to obtain waveform, nail polish, additional room light entering the inside of the probe, and being a smoker, to just name a few (Smoking increases carbon monoxide levels in the blood and the pulse oximeter cannot distinguish between carbon monoxide and oxygen and thus giving a false high oxygen saturation level.)

Also, patients tend to focus on "the number" and not the bigger picture. The bigger picture is themselves. What is normal for one person may not be normal for someone else. For example, a COPD patient's body oxygen level will adjust to a lower oxygen level over time, which will become their new normal. For the pulmonary fibrosis patient, the resting result is not as important as the recovery time.

And then there is the hospice field nurse who will call and tell me their patient's oxygen level is 96% or 87%, and I will ask, "On oxygen?"

And the response I will receive will be

"Oh, I don't know." or "Yes."

"OK, what type and how much?"

"Oh, I don't know."

I really want to ask them why they call me with useless information. Is that 96% or 87% on room air (21% oxygen) or have they turned their oxygen flow up to 10 LPM when it should be 2 LPM? Was that result obtained during rest or activity, were they using their PAP (Positive Airway Pressure) unit, is the oxygen delivered via concentrator or liquid? Or numerous other items that must be placed in context with the reported pulse-oximetry number to accurately assess the patient.

These pulse oximetry devices are mass-produced from cheap plastic and inexpensive components. However, they have a place if the patient understands their correct usage, limitations, and where they fit into their overall picture of health monitoring. As simple as a device may look, it is not just a matter of placing it on a finger and running with a number.

When a therapist does a six-minute pulse oximetry on a patient, it has separate parts of a testing protocol to measure a patient's oxygen requirements—with and without oxygen, as well as at rest and with exertion.

Part one starts with obtaining a patient's room air baseline pulse oximetry oxygen level. This baseline is done when the patient is at rest without oxygen. If the patient's oxygen level is 89% or above, the testing procedure continues to part two. If the oxygen level is 88% or lower, the testing skips to part three, as the patient automatically qualifies for oxygen.

Part two is done if the patient's baseline reading is at or above 89%. The patient is then asked to walk (or do other forms of exertion, arm lifts, etc.) until the reading drops to or below 88%, or if the heart rate increases by twenty beats per minute. This exercise can last up to six minutes, with the therapist noting pulse oximetry results and heart rate at one-minute intervals. If the patient's oxygen level drops to 88% or below with exertion, the patient qualifies for oxygen and the testing continues with part three.

Part three starts with obtaining a patient's baseline with oxygen in use. The patient is placed on low-flow oxygen via nasal cannula, usually at two liters per minute (written as 2 LPM). With the patient at rest, an oxygen level by pulse oximetry is obtained, and the oxygen flow is titrated for an oxygen level at or above 90%. This establishes a patient's supplemental oxygen requirement at rest.

Part four: The patient walks or performs other exercises for up to six minutes while maintaining an oxygen level of 90% or higher, with the therapist taking pulse oximetry readings at one-minute intervals and adjusting the oxygen as needed. This part of the test establishes a patient's supplemental oxygen requirement with exertion.

Please note: This is not a "How-To". This is only for informational purposes because this procedure has the potential to cause harm or death, and there are numerous factors and variations of this procedure that can only be determined appropriate and safe by the therapist at the time of testing.

## Bedside Spirometry

Bedside or simple spirometry is one part of a complete pulmonary function test (PFT). The handheld type of bedside spirometry looks at two parts of lung function:

Forced Vital Capacity (FVC): This maneuver measures how much air you can forcefully blow out in one breath.

FEV1 stands for Forced Expiratory Volume: This measures how much of the FVC air was blown out in the first second.

A bedside spirometry is a quick, easy, and inexpensive way to preliminarily detect a lung condition that may or may not need further testing, such as doing a complete PFT. Additionally, it is a tool used to monitor decline, as with a hospice patient.

The results of any type of testing, whether simple spirometry or a complete PFT, heavily depend on patient effort, coordination, understanding of the testing procedure, and the competency of the therapist administering the test. Pulmonary Function Testing is a specialized branch of respiratory therapy with credentials (CPFT or RPFT) and requires additional education.

A patient's family stated to me that a new hospice therapist visited the patient and had the patient do bedside spirometry. This patient was diagnosed with muscular dystrophy and was ventilator-dependent. His use of the ventilator was in a supportive AVAP mode via a full face mask, with 24/7 bedside care provided privately by the family. The therapist removed the patient from the ventilator and had him perform bedside spirometry. When the family asked the results, the therapist responded, "I don't know. I don't even know what the numbers mean." If that therapist did not know what the numbers meant, how did she/he know if the maneuver was performed correctly and consistently, they would not? And then to report those results is mind-boggling and malpractice. Not to mention testing a ventilator-dependent patient. Useless and dangerous.

Peak inspiratory flow

(PIF) measurement. As its name implies, this test measures the peak inspiratory flow generated during one inhaled breath. This testing is done on those patients who use dry powder inhalers such as Spiriva, Advair, Breo, or numerous others available on the market. It is performed with a tube-like device with an internal slide bar. The slide bar will correlate to a corresponding number printed outside the device, representing the inhaled flow expressed in liters per minute. It has an adjustable dial to vary the resistance level.

The maneuver is performed by having the patient exhale completely and then inhale as quickly and deeply as they would when using their dry powder inhaler.

This test does not measure a patient's response to the medication; it measures their ability to extract the medication from the dispensing device. Dispensing devices have different variations of resistance levels, and it takes effort to breathe in the medication from the dispenser.

Medications such as Advair are contained within a Diskus dispenser, Breo and Incruse are within an Ellipta, and Spiriva is dispensed from a handihaler. The manufacturers of such devices have guidelines for obtaining optimum flow rates from the patient for optimal medication retrieval from the dispenser.

The respiratory therapist was responsible when we instituted a program to evaluate a patient's respiratory health. However, this responsibility was later turned over to the nurses to perform. The problem with this transfer of responsibility is that the respiratory therapist is specially trained to assess respiratory function in the patient. With a small group of respiratory therapists, there was consistency in the testing of the patient and the accuracy of the results.

The team nurses were already overloaded with their duties and assessments of the patient. Because it was viewed as "RT duty," they had little interest in conducting the testing, let alone knowing whether or not the results were accurate.

Nurses would call while in the patient's home, asking for instructions on how to perform the test. One nurse took the device and an instruction sheet to a patient's home and asked the patient to help her assemble the device and tell her how the test should be done.

The nurses would send the results to the medical secretary to compile, and a copy of the email would be sent to me to review the results.

The results were to be reported as three separate numbers.

The first number would represent the patient's inspiratory flow effort when using an inhaler device without any resistance (Free Flow).

The second number would represent the patient's inspiratory flow effort with resistance equal to that of a Diskus (Advair) or Ellipta (Breo, Incruse) dispensing device.

The third number would represent the patient's inspiratory flow effort with resistance equal to that of the Handihaler (Spiriva Medication) dispensing device.

Knowing that the Free Flow result would be the highest number, followed by the Diskus/Ellipta and finally the Handihaler, a report of the numbers would follow a logical sequence.

For example, a report of the results would look something like 95/60/30.

The 95 indicates the inspiratory flow without any resistance.

The 60 indicates the inspiratory flow of the Diskus or Ellipta.

The 30 indicates the inspiratory flow of the Handihaler.

I would receive reports such as:

"The PIF was 10. Should I report it to anyone else?"
My response was that the nurse should check the patient for a pulse.

"PIF result 55. The policy says to ask for an RT consult. Can I refill her Advair?" *55 of what? Free Flow, Diskus, Ellipta?

"I didn't do a free flow. I'm sorry. This was my first time using this thing."

I brought this information to the corporate medical director and the chief clinical and compliance officer on numerous occasions regarding the nurses' lack of training and interest in performing the procedure correctly. With the amount of nursing turnover, these results would never be accurate.

Like the PFT testing, this test was also heavily dependent on patient effort, coordination, understanding of the testing procedure, as well as the state of the patient at the time of the visit. Like everyone else, the hospice patient will have good and bad days; unfortunately, for someone in this stage of their life, the bad days will be more pronounced. Without consistency of the same clinician testing the patient each month, there was no way to know if the results this month aligned with last month's results.

So now that you have a basic understanding of peak inspiratory flow testing, you know more than the nurses who do the testing. And you must be wondering why this is important.

This program originally came about due to increased hospital readmissions of our hospice patients. We needed to know if we were managing our patient's symptoms appropriately. Our test pilot included a random sample of twenty patients. Of those twenty patients, only half could retrieve the optimal dose of medication from the dispensing device by generating the inspiratory flow recommended by the manufacturer. Half the patients prescribed dry powder inhalers could not extract the medication from the dispenser. The medication they thought they were taking never left the dispenser.

If a patient cannot retrieve the medication from the dispenser, the medicine stays in the dispenser, not in the patient. At this point, these inhalers would be discontinued, and other types of medications would be prescribed.

However, as with any good deed, corporate America can turn it into money. When the bean counters noticed how much money was being saved by discontinuing the inhalers, the program seemed to have taken that money over patient care, which is why the nurses were now doing the testing. If the nurses were doing the testing and getting false low readings or reporting that the patient could not do something when the nurse did not know how to do the test, the patient's medications were discontinued. At an average cost of $300 per month for each dry powder inhaler, and with some patients having more than one inhaler, you can see where this program was headed.

I now regret any involvement in establishing this program. What I saw as a way to help our patients have a better quality of life appears to have turned into a way for others to better their quality of life. Sad and disappointing. Another piece of tint fell from my rose-colored glasses.

*GOLD Initiative*

The Global Initiative for Chronic Obstructive Lung Disease (GOLD) is a group of doctors, scientists, and other health professionals from all over the world who work together to share ideas, raise awareness of COPD, and improve prevention and treatment for patients worldwide. The classifications are:

GOLD 1 Mild FEV1 <80% of predicted

GOLD 2 FEV1 Moderate 50% to 80% of predicted

GOLD 3 Severe FEV1 30–50% of predicted

GOLD 4 Very Severe FEV1 < 30% of predicted

Modified British

The Modified British Medical Research Council relates to other measures of health status and predicts future mortality risk with a questionnaire, then classifies patients with shortness of breath (SOB) with a "Grade".

Grade 0 with strenuous exercise

Grade 1 Hurrying on level ground or walking up a hill

Grade 2 Stopping for breath when walking at your own pace on level ground

Grade 3 Stop for breath after a walk of 100 meters or a few minutes on level ground.

Grade 4 Too breathless to leave the house or breathless dressing/undressing.

These classification systems are used together with an assessment grid to include an exacerbation of symptoms.

This multi prong approach remains vital for the diagnosis, prognostication and consideration of other important therapeutic options for the COPD patient.

*Road Trip Home*
(From page 136).

COPD

Chronic Obstructive Pulmonary Disease (COPD) is a catch-all phrase that includes emphysema and bronchitis, among others, in which there is a ventilatory defect.

The airways and air sacs become less flexible, thus trapping air, and the patient has trouble getting air in and out of the lungs.

ILD

Interstitial Lung Disease is a catch-all phrase that includes Idiopathic Pulmonary Fibrosis, Sarcoidosis, and Asbestosis, among others, is an oxygenation defect.

In the most simple description of the lungs, the lungs can be described as five clusters of grapes. It is in these clusters (lobes) of grapes (alveoli) that the gas exchange process happens.

The respiratory system starts at the back of the throat with the trachea extending down the front inside part of the neck into the chest area. At about mid-nipple line, the trachea divides into two airways, one to the right and one to the left.

The airway to the right subdivides into three smaller airways that now start the three lobes. While the airway on the left subdivides into only two lobes to accommodate the heart.

Once these airways start in the lobe section of the lungs, the airways become smaller and smaller until they end in a vast cluster of grapes (alveoli). On average, there are 500 million alveoli in an adult with a surface area of almost 40 times greater than the body's outer surface, making the lungs one of the largest organs in the body.

It is here, at the alveoli, that gas exchange takes place. The air breathed in travels through the lungs, which have a network of smaller airways into the alveoli. Once in the alveoli, the gas mixture crosses the lung membrane into the bloodstream. The gases are then transported to the tissue site and used. The cells at the tissue site use the oxygen from the inhaled gas mixture, and a byproduct of the oxygen usage is carbon dioxide. The carbon dioxide is then transported back to the lungs where it is exhaled through the breathing process. **There are many factors that affect this extremely complex system.

Then, next to alveoli in the lining of the lung interstitium. It is this lining that has inflammation, scarring, and thickening. Instead of this lining being the thickness of a piece of paper, it is now the thickness of a nickel. This example is for visual comparison only.

This thickening increases the time it takes for oxygen to diffuse from the lung into the capillary blood flow. In addition to the actual thickening, the cells are also tightly compacted from the inflammation and scarring. This is what keeps the oxygen from passing from the airways in the lungs to the blood as freely as it should.

Patients with Interstitial Lung Disease (ILD) can keep their oxygen levels up if they do not move AND they are on high-flow liquid oxygen. Any type of movement, even moving from the bed to the bedside commode, can be too much. Once their oxygen level drops, it is very hard and it takes a long time to bring their oxygen level back into a "normal" range. known as "slow recovery." For these patients, it is always better for them to keep up with their oxygen demands than to catch up. You never want to put a patient with ILD in a catch-up phase. That could be deadly.

*Death Through Chemistry*
(From page 159)

Medication safety standards within the healthcare field are extensive and, if followed appropriately, could and would save hundreds of thousands of lives each year from medication errors. According to the World Health Organization (WHO) 3/2018, "There is a 1 in a million chance of a person being harmed while traveling by plane. In comparison, there is a 1 in 300 chance of a patient being harmed during health care. Industries with a perceived higher risk, such as the aviation and nuclear industries, have a much better safety record than health care.

John Hopkins University released a study in 2016 that was conducted over eight years of data analyzing medical death rates. They concluded that more than 250,000 deaths per year are due to medical errors in the U.S.

Consider this: according to this study, 250,000 people die each year as a result of medication errors.

The prestigious British Medical Journal (BMJ) (published without interruption since 1840) is an international peer-reviewed medical journal which published these findings. Significantly, these statistics would put medication errors as the third leading cause of death in the U.S., only surpassed by heart disease (#1) and cancer (#2). These findings push Chronic Respiratory Disease to the #4 spot.

The John Hopkins team of Martin Makary and Michael Daniel, who authored this study, are advocating for updated criteria for classifying deaths on death certificates.

Incident rates for deaths directly attributable to medical care gone awry haven't been recognized in any standardized method for collecting national statistics, says Martin Makary, M.D., M.P.H., professor of surgery at the Johns Hopkins University School of Medicine and an authority on health reform.

"The medical coding system was designed to maximize billing for physician services, not to collect national health statistics, as it is currently being used."

Meaning, by categorizing and calculating national mortality derived from billing codes, is inherently flawed. At that time, it was under-recognized that diagnostic errors, medical mistakes, and the absence of safety nets could result in someone's death, and because of that, medical errors were unintentionally excluded from national health statistics," says Makary.

Makary and Daniel's conclusions are not without their detractors.

Two researchers, Kaveh G. Shojania, a scientist at Sunnybrook Research Institute, and Mary Dixon-Woods, a Rand professor of health services researcher, challenged the John Hopkins study in their analysis, also published in the BMJ. Citing that the methodology was "precarious" and that, on average, only 700,000 deaths occur in hospitals each year, this would mean that medical error is responsible for one-third of hospital deaths.Which, in itself, is hard to believe. Just as most deaths do not involve a medical error, most medical errors do not produce death, but they can still produce substantial morbidity, costs, suffering, and distress.

The reported numbers could be even higher than the data suggests. Patients who receive medications are not only in the hospital; they are in Assisted Living Facilities (ALF), Nursing Homes, Outpatient Centers, and at home, just to name a few.

How many of these places have medication errors that they report? Or that the caregiver actually recognizes the mistake?

Is it staff circumventing safety protocols to keep up with all the demands placed on them by organizations cutting staffing levels to the bare minimum? Are there systemic problems or a lack of procedures for coordination of care between healthcare providers and insurance companies?

While I can see both sides of this argument, medical errors are almost completely unrecognized as a cause of death, whether directly or indirectly responsible, and this is where at least all the authors seem to agree.

Patient safety goals include the following when administering medications or before performing any procedure:

The ideal patient

The right medication

The right dose

The right site

The right time

The right route

The right reason

However, this only addresses one aspect of the process.

And while I am on this subject, let me add that medical errors happen anywhere there is a patient, a caregiver, medications, equipment, procedures to be done, pharmacies to fill prescriptions, doctors to write prescriptions, and this list could go on and on.

While you may feel safe from such a tragedy, you are not. When it comes to medical errors, everyone is at risk. It does not matter if you are rich and famous or poor and unknown. It does not matter if you are white, black, or brown, nor what nationality you are. Let me throw a few names out there.

Prince, Elvis, Michael Jackson, Bill Paxton, Joan Rivers, King George V, and many more, known and unknown, have become victims of medical mistakes or careless doctors, institutes, pharmacies, and yes, even newspaper deadlines. No pun intended.

*King George V (June 3, 1865 – January 20, 1936) - The King's physician, Lord Dawson of Penn, wrote in his dairy, that he hastened the King's death by injecting him with morphine and cocaine. The reason? So that the King's death would be before the deadline of the morning paper. In 1986, the contents of Dawson's diary were made public for the first time, in which he clearly acknowledged what he had done and was described by a medical reviewer in 1994 as an arrogant "convenience killing".

## Useful Links

Find your State's Congressman or Senator, view pending legislation, Live video feed, Committee reports and schedules, and much more.
congress.gov

Office of the Inspector General - Submit a complaint, search website for healthcare fraud, whistleblower protection, enforcement actions. This website is a must view.
OIG.hhs.gov

Marsha Joiner - Talkshow Host: Betrayed By Hospice. An in-depth look at hospice with personal accounts from families who have lost their loved ones by hospice, as well as other healthcare crisis such as elder abuse, guardianship take-overs, organ donor issues and pending healthcare legislation. (In conjunction with TS Radio Network and Marti Oakley)
BlogTalkRadio.com

Washington Post Newspaper - Search 'Hospice Neglect'
washingtonpost.com

New York Times - Search 'Hospice Fraud'
nytimes.com

Kasem Cares - The mission of Kasem Cares and the Kasem Coalition is to eliminate all forms of elder abuse, including isolation, through education and awareness, as well as support of social change and legislative action. *Taken from their website.
kasemcares.org

Healthcare Advocacy and Leadership Organization - HALO strives to protect, support, and advocate for medically vulnerable persons without discrimination based on race, religion, age, disability, sex, or sexual orientation. *Taken from their website.
halovoice.org

"Choice" is an illusion - A non-profit corporate opposed to assisted suicide and euthanasia, worldwide.
choiceillusion.org

## About The Author

Michelle's career in respiratory therapy took off in the mid-1980s when she graduated with a degree in respiratory science. She later earned national credentials as a Registered Respiratory Therapist (RRT) and Certified Pulmonary Function Technologist (CPFT) and continued her education with a B.S. in Health Sciences. Additionally, Michelle is a Certified Smoking Cessation Counselor and a Certified Paralegal specializing in Trial Litigation.

Throughout her career, Michelle has worked in various areas of respiratory science, including neonatal, pediatrics, adult, emergency, trauma, surgery, intensive care, flight, and home healthcare. She has served as an ethics board member for four major hospitals in the Tampa Bay Area and as an adjunct professor at a local college.

Michelle has provided care and worked with numerous high-profile celebrities and politicians, including a Governor, a State Senator, and a former Vice President of the United States. She received an employee recognition award from a prestigious hospital in the Tampa Bay area for her dedication to patient excellence.

Michelle has been featured in magazines and radio shows for her expertise in pulmonary rehabilitation and her insights into the decline of the healthcare system. In her free time, she enjoys playing golf, creating digital art, and making junk journals when her beloved fur babies permit it. Her bucket list includes landing and taking off from an aircraft carrier and holidaying in the Maldives.

In her book, "Killing For Profit - The Dark Side of Hospice," Michelle shares her incredible journey and experiences as a respiratory therapist, offering a unique perspective on the healthcare system. As a respiratory therapist, Michelle has dedicated her life to helping patients with respiratory-compromised conditions, and her book is a testament to her passion and commitment to her profession.

To understand Michelle, you need to know her mom, Lilian Rosa. Lilian was born in 1931 in England. At the age of 15, Lilian was determined to be accepted into the local nursing school. However, the infirmary would not allow admission to nursing school until the age of 17. This did not prevent Lilian from going to the infirmary almost every day for the next year and a half. Meanwhile, everyone in the infirmary got to know Lilian.

Then, at the age of 16 and a half, Lilian was allowed to help the other nurses. When she turned 17, Lilian was allowed to enter the three-year nursing program. Talking to Lilian now, who turned 89 in March 2020, those years were some of her fondest memories.

Shortly after the war, Lilian moved to America and was hired by a surgeon to be his scrub nurse. Lilian worked in his office, toured the hospital with him, and assisted him in surgery.

Lilian's children had a childhood full of all kinds of animals. Their mother even brought home an owl that had been shot out of one eye by a BB gun. Lilian brought it back to health.

So when you look at Lilian's determination to become a nurse and then to excel in her profession and her love of animals, Michelle is cut from the same cloth.

Be the voice of the voiceless.
Adopt a family member, don't buy a pet.

## Michelle Young Doers

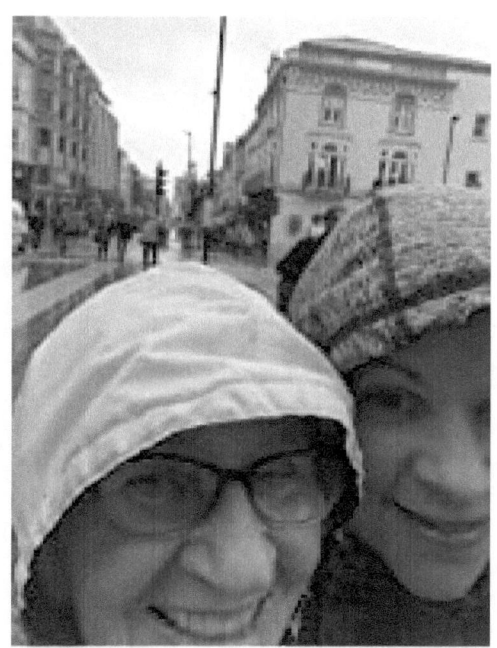

www.ingramcontent.com/pod-product-compliance
Lightning Source LLC
Chambersburg PA
CBHW021814170526
45157CB00007B/2591